Schizophrenia
or
Spirit Possession

Mike Williamson

TRICORN
BOOKS

Schizophrenia
or
Spirit Possession
Mike Williamson

Text © Mike Williamson unless otherwise stated
Design © 131 Design

ISBN: 978-1-909660-37-3

British Library Cataloguing in Publication Data.
A catalogue record for this book is available from the British Library.

Published 2014 by
Tricorn Books
131 High Street
Old Portsmouth
PO1 2HW
www.tricornbooks.co.uk

Printed and bound in the UK

Schizophrenia
or
Spirit Possession

I'd like to thank Vanessa for the support, help and patience that she has shown me while proof-reading this book; for keeping me on the right track and the words of encouragement. Thank you and Danny for all the work you have done in our circle. Thanks to Dan, from Tricorn Books for help in creating the front cover, and for formatting and editing this book. And those whose stories have been told.

Contents

Preface

Since writing my first book, *Working in the Realms of Spirit*, the interest I received inspired me to write this book to explain my findings in more detail about spirit and spirit interference: there is more to spirit than haunted houses.

Over the years I have met some wonderful and interesting people from all walks of life, some of whom were diagnosed with mental problems or psychological problems, when it was clear they were receiving thoughts and feelings that weren't theirs. I am not a doctor and have no medical training, but as a medium I was aware of the thoughts and feelings coming from the spirit world. As I was developing my mediumistic abilities, I had first-hand experience of the different ways discarnate spirit could impact our daily lives. Budding mediums sit in development circles where we learn to understand how spirit is communicating with us. There are awareness circles which are open to anyone who wishes to attend and for the beginner who is maybe seeing or hearing things. This circle is so we can be trained to recognise information coming from spirit and when it is our own thoughts. There is also a closed circle where only those invited may attend. In the closed circle, the same people commit to sitting every week; it is for more advanced development and specialising in different forms of mediumship. Circles are run by more experienced mediums who are able to help and explain what is happening and how to present the information that is received from the spirit world. In any of these circles the budding medium may be introduced to one of their guides or guardian angels who work with them from the spirit world. Everyone has guides, but unless a person is developing, they will not need to be aware of them.

Many of the people I visited experienced or heard noises and bangs in the night as though things were being moved. Some were getting thoughts and feelings, but no tangible experiences. It was clear to me what was happening, although the individuals thought they were going mad or having a breakdown. Some had been diagnosed as mentally ill and put on drugs which subdued their awareness, but this wasn't always the answer as they were still troubled.

My aim as a medium is to help people and through time and experience this has naturally progressed into researching psychosis and some of its causes. This book is about my findings, and includes some case histories that I dealt with, in conjunction with our closed circle, which consists of Vanessa, Danny and myself. You will see in the research that psychosis is not always the problem and the case histories will demonstrate how I was able to help some of those who were being interfered with from the spirit realms.

Schizophrenia, Multiple Personality Disorder, Dissociative Identity Disorder and Bi-Polar Disorder are all psychotic illnesses that can also be associated with spirit interference. Each case has to be investigated separately, as no two are the same, and it would be irresponsible to say that all of the above are caused by spirit interference. The brain does malfunction and sometimes there may be other underlying causes. Most of the time drugs are prescribed in these cases to treat the symptoms - not the causes. In these situations it can be difficult to separate interference from physical malfunction. The prescribed drugs can alter the chemicals in the brain and also have side-effects that can distort the original symptoms until there is no way back from the situation the person finds themselves in. To give you an example, I suffer from Parkinson's disease and one of the symptoms is an uncontrollable shaking of the limbs: one of the side-effects of the drugs I am prescribed is trembling of the limbs. The medical profession can prescribe me other drugs to control the trembling, but to take them would give me other side-effects that are less pleasant than my limb-shaking. In the same way, the drugs that are given for psychosis can be debilitating and can change the whole way of life for the patient and not in a good way. Some who we were unable to help were taking so many drugs to counteract the side-effects of their main drug that it would be difficult to say to what extent the adverse reactions to the medicine were the underlying cause.

Introduction

Over the past 35 years working as a medium, it has become obvious to me that some 'mental illnesses' aren't what they seem to be. We are more than the physical body: there is a spiritual side to us that is not always obvious. The spirit world can and does interact - and sometimes interfere - with our daily lives. The medical profession and medical science doesn't always appreciate the interference that we can get from those who have passed on. They don't accept the possibility that we can be affected by discarnate spirit, because most don't accept that life continues in another dimension.

There is a lack of understanding about the brain and the mind - one is physical and the other is spiritual, connected by our life-force. The brain is the mechanical part, which deals with the everyday functions of the body. The mind deals with thoughts and emotions and is the receptacle of all our experiences. It is the mind that can be influenced by the thoughts of those in the spirit world and most of the time these thoughts are from our loved ones. Sometimes it is a memory of times gone by, or a feeling of not being alone. Most people will not necessarily recognise these thoughts as coming from those who have passed and think them their own. The mind can be influenced by anyone in spirit if they wish to; they only have to direct a thought and the mind will sometimes pick up these stray thoughts. Most of those who get lost do so usually because of their beliefs, or because they don't know they have died. Though they are lost they are safe, yet often confused as to what has happened to them, especially if they die unexpectedly. There are also those who know exactly what has happened and some will take advantage of the ability to influence those on the earth plane. Most people pass over with no problems and are met and cared for by their loved ones, but if just a few get lost then - over the years - that can add up to a lot of lost souls.

A lot of people who pass through drug or alcohol addiction and many who are in hospital, have been taking prescribed drugs to ease their pain. They are initially no more aware when they pass than they were before they passed: it can take time to adjust and sometimes they will need help from their loved ones in the spirit world, who gather round at the time of passing to help

1

them. Some of those who take street drugs and overdose will expect the drug to wear off after a while and - if addicted - will go looking for another fix. They can be attracted to people on the earth plane who are addicts or taking prescribed drugs. In their desperation to get another high, they may try to influence the person on the earth plane to take more and more drugs.

The following shows how people are being misled by medical science. Schizophrenia, Bi-Polar Disorder, (BPD) Multiple Personality Disorder, (MPD) and Dissociative Identity Disorder (DID) are not diseases. I will show you why I believe this to be true. MPD and DID are the same thing, DID being the new name for people with multiple personalities. Psychiatry is not dealing with the root cause of people's mental aberrations because they are looking in the wrong place. They should consider the mind as part of the soul, and the brain as part of the physical body; how the mind can be subject to outside interference by other souls and not affected by disease or chemical imbalance like the brain. They also need to ask themselves why administering drugs will not relieve the suffering of the soul, but can cause malfunction in the brain.

Most psychiatrists use hypnosis in their attempt to help their clients. This is much like the trance state that mediums go into when channelling discarnate spirits. How can any psychiatrist know when they are talking to spirit if they don't believe in the spirit realms, or consider the possibility? All the above disorders are to do with the psyche, which is the mind - not the brain. Another name for the psyche is the soul. How can they psychoanalyse someone when they aren't considering the soul? I have included some case histories to show how we have dealt with some people who have been diagnosed as psychotic. Sometimes, if the individual has not had spirit interference for too long, we have been able to resolve their problems quickly. Sometimes it takes time and re-education to help people to understand what they are experiencing. Sometimes we are unable to help, as they either don't understand or are not determined enough to assert their mind to get things under control. There are also those we can't help because they have been taking drugs for too long and it has affected their mind-set. We will see that some of the people we visited don't have the will or focus to fight off the spiritual attacks.

The problem initially was not their brain malfunctioning, but their unconscious mind being influenced by discarnate spirits. I was determined to help those that I could. Some of the people I have helped kindly agreed to allow me to tell their stories.

Most of the spirits were just looking for help, and weren't aware they had died. Some were in pain and, not realising they had died, continued to feel the discomfort after their passing. This caused them distress and while trying to attract attention, they inadvertently transmitted their feelings to the person they were attached to, who thought it was their own pain.

Through my years of development, I had come to the conclusion that the brain and the mind are two separate things, the mind being part of the soul or spirit and the brain an organ of the physical body. Both work together, but in very different ways.

Sometimes the mind, or subconscious, is more accessible than at other times, usually because of heightened sensitivity caused by big events in people's lives. This might be, for example, strong emotions felt when someone passes or relationships break up. When this happens, people can become aware of the spirit realms unknowingly. Because they are not used to receiving this information, they will usually think it is part of their physical world and treat it accordingly. This is why mediums take time to develop their psychic gifts. They have to learn to recognise which world they are tuning in to.

I will attempt to show that brain disorders are organic and physical, while the mind is energy and not subject to disease or malfunction like the brain. I will show how I met people who had been diagnosed with a mental illness without taking the spirit realms into consideration. I intend to show in the case histories how some of the people I met were troubled by discarnate spirits and not mental illness. I look primarily at schizophrenia but also include DID, MPD and BPD from both the medical and spiritual point of view. I will show how the media and medical science mislead people about drugs and how they are still guessing at the reasons why people have these complaints; and how many psychiatrists still haven't accepted the fact that the mind and the brain are two separate, but integrated, parts of the human reality.

I will show how disease of the brain is not disease of the mind and how hallucinations are more likely to come from the mind -

or soul - rather than the brain, unless drug-induced or there is a physical brain malfunction. I also look at how the brain, because it's so closely linked to the mind, can be easily influenced by discarnate spirits; how this influence is not always intentional, (but there are those who will invade for personal reasons); and how I have helped people to overcome the interference from the spirit world.

The cases in this book are true: only the names and places have been changed to protect their privacy. I would also like to express my thanks to those who gave permission for their stories to be told in the hope that others won't suffer as they did.

Our Circle

There are three of us in our circle: Vanessa, Danny and me, and between us we have many different mediumistic abilities.

We sit in a circle because, when developing would-be mediums and more advanced mediums, a circle has no end and no beginning. We also sit in a circle so we can see everyone and so that some of the more experienced can observe spirits when they come to communicate. A circle is easier to protect from outside influences by unwanted spirits and we are able to build spiritual energy which helps the spirits we are working with to communicate. This spiritual energy also helps the sitters to raise their vibrations to a higher level to make communication easier.

I have been a medium for 35 years and use my senses to perceive spirits. I have been helping lost souls for more than 30 years to find peace. I am a clairsentient and trance medium and run development circles to teach others how to communicate with the spirit world. I also teach trance and do demonstrations of mediumship in the local spiritualist churches.

Vanessa has been aware of spirit for about 30 years. She is a clairsentient medium, healer and holistic therapist. Vanessa's skills enhance our circle and she is able to explain things to the people we meet in a way that they can understand.

Danny is a trance medium who has been working in that capacity for the past five years. He is also developing his clairvoyant gifts and healing to enhance his rescue work.

We have visited many houses where spirits have been active

and we've been able to explain and help people understand what's happening. We have also had the privilege of helping lost souls who are causing distress to the families who live in the houses, to find their way home. Most of the lost souls are unknown to the inhabitants of the houses. They are attracted to properties and people for many different reasons. If one of the people in the house is sensitive to the spirit world this can attract lost or confused souls in the hope they will get help. These lost souls are unaware of the spirit realms because their focus is still on the earth plane, which is why they are lost.

What are we?

Each person is part of an eternal energy that we call 'spirit' or the 'godhead'. Spirit is the life-force, the vital force that characterises the person as being alive. We are spirit in a physical body, which is alien to our normal state, which is energy. When we are born into the physical world, we initially retain our spiritual awareness. Gradually, as we become more aware of our physical surroundings, our spiritual reality fades into our subconscious. We then become dependent on the sights and sounds of our physical reality. We still have our spiritual essence, but our focus is on the obvious stimulation from our physical surroundings. Different types of spirit may be called God, Angels, Guardian Angels, Guides or Ascended Masters. There are many names that can be used, depending on one's teachings and understanding. I work closely with my guides and have been encouraged to write this book to show there are other possibilities for the cause of psychosis. Of course, I am aware that the brain does malfunction just like the rest of the body. But the mind is energy and part of the soul where we store our experiences and is not subject to physical diseases.

Our spiritual body is energy, more commonly known as the aura or astral body that surrounds our physical body: it can be subject to influence from the spirit world. This is because, in the same way that our physical body can be affected by material things, our astral body can be affected by other energy bodies in the spirit world. Just as our physical body is stimulated by sight, sound, touch, taste and smell in the physical world, the influences from the spirit world can often be mistaken for physical stimuli. The brain and mind are interconnected by our life-force and the mind is the receptacle of all our experiences. These experiences are stored from our earlier lives and times in the spirit world and make up the sum total of who we are. If, as I believe, we are here to gain knowledge and to experience life in the physical, then it stands to reason we will need to have more than one life. How would I know what life is like from a woman's point of view if I had never been a woman? Spirit is genderless, so can be born as male or female. We will also spend time in the spirit world between lives, gaining more understanding. As we continue

6

through our current life, we continue to store more experiences.

The brain is a physical organ and is stimulated by our awareness of the physical world around us. But the soul or mind is stimulated by the spirit world and is connected by our subconscious to our brain. The brain runs the physical body and is affected by the rigours of the world around us. It is subject to all sorts of malfunctions, which can be caused by chemicals, drugs or even the environment we are in. The brain also deteriorates through aging and brain diseases such as Alzheimer's, multiple sclerosis and Parkinson's disease, all of which are degenerative and take their toll.

The mind, however, is not subject to any disease or chemical imbalances as it is not an organ of the body, but part of the soul or spirit.

It is important to realise that we are living in two places at once, the physical world and the spiritual, which gives us a dual existence. The spirit world interconnects with the physical world and although it occupies the same space, it vibrates at a different frequency and is therefore unfortunately unseen by most people. The earthly plane is much denser than the spirit plane, but is as real to spirit as our world is to us. Once this is accepted, then proper attention will be paid to the influences from the spirit world. Most people are unaware of this dual existence but will accept there is something more than this life. Since mankind could think, he has accepted the possibility that life goes on after death of the physical form. It's not a coincidence that religions have been based on this concept since the beginning of time.

Schizophrenia

Some of the people I met who were experiencing spiritual problems also had a history of mental problems. Others were on anti-depressants or visiting a psychiatrist and there were a few who had been in and out of mental institutions and were taking prescribed drugs. I was unable to help most of these people because either they had become reliant on the drugs they were taking or their symptoms were the effect of the drugs.

Others had even undergone electroconvulsive therapy without any significant change taking place. I became increasingly dissatisfied with my approach to their problem, as I knew it was spiritual. Most of these people were living on their own and were isolated from families and friends. Because of the different treatments and drugs they had taken, they didn't have the strength of mind to stand up to their spiritual interference, or have the support of family and friends.

Because they had been diagnosed by a psychiatrist, they had accepted the diagnosis without question. Once they were taking the drugs, their brain was affected. I was unable to help them to understand that the problem might now be a chemical imbalance, and that their brain may have been damaged by the drugs. Even if they stopped taking the medications prescribed, there was no certainty that their brain would return to normal. I had undergone similar interference; I understood their problem. It was fortunate that I knew it was spiritual interference that I was getting and so I never resorted to medical help. I knew that if I couldn't help them to understand how to control their emotions, they would be plagued with interference for the rest of their lives. I was aware that the medical profession had criteria which stated that if you heard voices, or saw people that others couldn't see, then you were suffering from hallucinations, and the only remedy they had was to pump you full of neuroleptic drugs. I found that those who had been taking the drugs for a while had come to depend on them and that the side effects could make things worse. They were taking one drug to counter the side-effects of another, until they had such a cocktail that there was no knowing what damage was being done to their brain. Not being a psychiatrist or a doctor, it's difficult say whether they were prescribed for schizophrenia or if there were other underlying conditions. But it was clear that all the people who were on these drugs had spirit interference. It's known that patients who have been taking neuroleptic drugs can have brain damage caused by the drugs prescribed. Drugs are given to treat the symptoms, not necessarily the cause, which can be spiritual. The drugs desensitise the brain (not the mind) by blocking the brain receptors, thereby weakening the link between brain and mind. So unfortunately there is nothing to be done for those people. On a more promising note, I was able to resolve the problems of those I have come in contact with (and there have been many) who were not taking drugs.

Schizophrenia, MPD, DID and BPD are all problems that can be confused with each other and therefore, according to the medical profession, it is difficult to accurately diagnose one from the other. If they considered them all to be part of the same problem, and took a spiritual point of view, they might have more of a chance of resolving them. Many of the drugs prescribed for the above can make the conditions worse, as it is not fully known how much damage is being done to the brain by these drugs. Two drugs that are often used are Thorazine, more commonly known as Chlorpromazine, and Resperdal, more commonly known as Risperidone. They are used to treat schizophrenia, BPD, MPD and DID and Risperidone is also used to treat children to relieve them of irritability. Why would you give a child such a powerful drug just because they're irritable? These drugs work by changing the effects and balance of chemicals in the brain.

Electroconvulsive Therapy (ECT) was used a lot in the early 1940s, the idea being to induce a seizure of the brain to try and reset the neural pathways. In those days they just used to strap people down and put two contacts - one on either side of the head - and shock them. The spasms that resulted from these electric shocks could and did cause broken bones when the patient's muscles went into spasm.

ECT is typically used nowadays to treat severe depression, but is also used for other mental illnesses like schizophrenia. During ECT, an electric current is briefly applied through the scalp to the brain, inducing a seizure.

They say ECT is one of the fastest ways to relieve symptoms in severely depressed and suicidal patients, or patients who suffer from mania or other mental illnesses. ECT is generally used as a last resort when severe depression is unresponsive to other forms of therapy, or when these patients pose a severe threat to themselves or others and it's dangerous to wait until medications take effect, which can be up to four weeks.

Nowadays they put patients under with a mild anaesthetic and give them a muscle relaxant so they don't tense up. The patient usually awakens a few minutes later not remembering the treatment or events surrounding it. They're often confused at first, but this confusion typically lasts for only a short period of time. ECT is usually given up to three times a week for two to four weeks. This is then followed by psychotherapy and medication. They say it's safe and among the most effective treatments available for depression. Yet Schizophrenia isn't depression, so why would they use it? They also say it may provide temporary improvement but that it has a high relapse rate.

As schizophrenia cannot be proven by pathology and medical science doesn't know what causes it, how can they class it as a mental illness?

What causes schizophrenia?

According to the scientists, schizophrenia is a complex disorder that does not have one single known cause.

There are four main theories that are thought by scientists to be the most likely explanation of schizophrenia, but these are not 100 percent proven and research into the causes of schizophrenia is still being conducted.

Genetics

Schizophrenia can run in families: if one or more close relatives has schizophrenia, the chances of developing it are increased. Schizophrenia itself is not inherited but rather a genetic predisposition to develop the illness. In cases of genetic predisposition, there is usually a factor that will trigger the person into developing schizophrenia, such as high levels of stress, life events, the environment, or even a viral infection.

Brain Chemistry

Although research into this area is not one hundred percent conclusive, there is much evidence to suggest that brain chemistry plays an important role in the development of schizophrenia. It is believed that chemical imbalances in the brain (particularly of the neurotransmitters, namely dopamine and glutamate) could be the cause of schizophrenic disorders.

Pregnancy and birth complications

It is thought by some scientific researchers that a viral infection during pregnancy, lack of nutrition to the foetus during pregnancy, or complications during birth can increase the baby's chance of developing schizophrenia in later life.

Brain abnormality

The use of neuroimaging has given doctors and researchers the opportunity to look at the brains of people with schizophrenia and other mental illnesses. What has been seen in the brains of schizophrenic patients are abnormalities in the structure of the brain (such as areas of the brain being too large or too small for example) and in the function of the brain, such as problems with the metabolism within the brain.

It is important to stress that not all schizophrenia patients have brain abnormalities and that not all people with brain abnormalities suffer from, or go on to develop, schizophrenia.

It's interesting to note that they think imbalances of dopamine could be a cause of Schizophrenia. I have Parkinson's disease, which is said to be caused by too little dopamine. Yet I can still communicate with spirit and have done for the past thirty-five years. They cannot find a cause for schizophrenia despite brain scans.

In other words they don't know, so maybe it's time to look at other avenues, such as the mind rather than the brain instead of blindly ignoring the possibility of outside interference from the spirit world.

Types of Schizophrenia

The different types of schizophrenia, as defined by the world's leading psychiatrists and neuroscientists, are:

Paranoid schizophrenia

Disorganised schizophrenia (Hebephrenic schizophrenia)

Catatonic schizophrenia

Residual schizophrenia

Schizoaffective disorder

Undifferentiated schizophrenia

Let's look at each of these types of schizophrenia with the spirit world in mind.

Paranoid schizophrenia: medical

People diagnosed as paranoid are very suspicious of others and often have elaborate theories of persecution at the root of their behaviour. Hallucinations and delusions are prominent.

Paranoid schizophrenia: spiritual

When spirit find someone who is receptive to their influences, they become very protective of their situation and don't want anyone to find out what they're doing. They give that person the feeling that they're being watched. This can cause the person who is being influenced to withdraw from social situations. Spirit can then have them to themselves in isolation. Why? So they can control them and continue to live through them on the earth plane. They will also give the individual thoughts and ideas that come from the mind of the spirit, planting scenarios in their mind which put them out of sync with the world around them. It's no wonder they think they are going out of their mind. A person does not have to be possessed to be affected by discarnate spirit, it can be just a subtle thought that intrudes on the mind. Not all spirits are like this: there are those who had degenerative brain disease or other illnesses that may cause disorientation. Or just spirits trying to make contact who know they have died, and who just wish to communicate. The medium can help here, in describing how the spirit is feeling. The medium's perspective is that the thoughts and feelings are from discarnate spirit instead of it being the medium's reality. Part of development is to learn to differentiate between a medium's own thoughts and feelings and those that emanate from spirit. The fact is that spirit do pass information on to the medium in a variety of ways - by seeing, thought, words, feelings, emotions and smell. If people are not aware that they might receive communication in this way, it's no wonder they get confused as to what is their own thought and what isn't. By talking to the spirit, a medium is able to explain their circumstances and help them to move on, to the next step on their spiritual pathway. Once this is done, the discarnate spirit will no longer affect the person, and the voices, thoughts, emotions and feelings will go away.

Disorganised schizophrenia (Hebephrenic schizophrenia): medical

People with disorganised schizophrenia have jumbled speech, and inappropriate changes to moods and emotions. Hallucinations are not normally present - similar to bi-polar disorder.

Disorganised schizophrenia: spiritual

This is where the spirit puts their own emotions and moods onto somebody else. This causes confusion and will play with their mind, so much so, they are unable to string two words together. This is much like a medium getting feelings and emotions from loved ones, sometimes emotions so strong that the medium has trouble speaking. By speaking to the discarnate spirit the medium is able to help them to overcome their emotions and understand they have died, helping them to find peace.

Catatonic schizophrenia: medical

Someone with catatonic schizophrenia may purposely adopt strange body positions, or establish unusual limb movements or facial expressions. This often results in a misdiagnosis of tardive dyskinesia (involuntary movement of the tongue and facial muscles). They are very withdrawn, negative and isolated, and are unable to control limbs and bodily movement, especially voluntary muscle action. They go from one extreme to the other - sometimes not able to speak, move or respond and there is a remarkable decrease in activity where all movement stops, as in catatonic daze. Other times they get overexcited or hyperactive, and occasionally copy sounds and movements around them, a condition sometimes referred to as catatonic excitement.

Catatonic schizophrenia: spiritual

In this case, the person is receiving negative thoughts and fears from spirit, usually unintentionally. They tend to isolate themselves from people around them because of how they are feeling, as others don't understand how and what's happening to them. This makes the individual feel alone and lethargic, and sometimes listless. Similar to the spirit of a loved one showing a medium how they felt towards the end of their life, when they were ill, or perhaps had a stroke, or Alzheimer's. The medium may actually experience the feelings, as well as being told what the communicator suffered with, and may also exhibit actions or habits peculiar to the communicator. By explaining to the spirit they have died, the medium is able to help them to understand they no longer have the ailments they had in life. Once the spirit understands this, it is able to move on and find peace. The person who was feeling the ailments, will no longer be affected.

Residual schizophrenia: medical

People with residual schizophrenia don't suffer from hallucinations, delusions or disorganised speech and behaviour. They don't have any interest or motivation in day-to-day living and can show eccentric behaviour and withdrawal from social activities.

Residual schizophrenia: spiritual

This is similar to the spiritual cause of catatonic schizophrenia, where a spirit is giving the feelings they experienced at certain times of their life - perhaps to describe the type of person they were, or perhaps an illness that made them feel tired or lethargic. They may have been depressed at some time in their life and are showing the medium how they felt, or they may be a lost spirit who has given up because they can't find the help they need. This can appear to be residual schizophrenia as categorised by the medical profession, when in actual fact they are being affected by the spirit. This is why it is so important to rule out spirit interference before prescribing medication. There are many mediums who don't see spirit, yet they work very well with feelings and emotions.

Schizoaffective disorder: medical

People with bi-polar mania, mixed mania schizophrenia and major depression may be diagnosed with schizoaffective disorder.

Schizoaffective disorder: spiritual

This is where somebody lives the feelings of the spirit, who will put their own sadness, fears and discomfort at maybe being lost and confused, onto someone else. They will feel the changes in mood as if they were their own. Again, this is similar to a medium picking up the feelings the loved ones are giving them, which is sometimes easier than the spirit trying to explain to the medium how they felt.

Undifferentiated schizophrenia: medical

Somebody who meets the general criteria for diagnosing schizophrenia but doesn't fit any of the above subtypes. Or, they may exhibit characteristics of more than one, without conforming to a particular set of diagnostic criteria.

Undifferentiated schizophrenia: spiritual

This is where a spirit who is experienced at communicating will use different ways to communicate. In most cases it just needs the medium to explain what has happened to the spirit - once they understand, they will happily take the next step on their journey. Medical professionals don't know what to do with these patients and until they accept that the mind is not part of the brain, they will always look in the wrong place for the cure.

According to experts, schizophrenia is an extremely complex illness and they find it difficult to establish its causes. The disorder exhibits a number of symptoms as it develops in its cycle and these are categorised into three main areas: positive, negative and cognitive.

Positive symptoms (called thus because they are easy to discern) include psychotic behaviour that would be uncharacteristic in healthy people. Individuals exhibiting these symptoms act illogically and the symptoms are inconsistent. They will experience hallucinations and they may see, hear or smell things others don't – the most common symptom is hearing voices. They may also experience delusions, which cause them to hold illogical beliefs, such as the conviction that someone is reading their mind or influencing how they behave. Positive symptoms will also include thought disorders, where somebody experiences disorganised thinking and is unable to express themselves logically or speak meaningful words. Movement disorders - 'catatonic behaviours' - are also common positive symptoms and they appear agitated in their body movements and may exhibit abnormal movement.

Unlike positive symptoms, negative symptoms are harder to distinguish from other conditions such as depression. They may include someone associating less or speaking little, being sad, or low in motivation. People experiencing these symptoms are often seen as lazy and may neglect basic issues such as hygiene.

Cognitive symptoms, just like negative symptoms, are those which make it difficult to tell the difference between schizophrenia and other illnesses, and are determined after performing tests. Someone exhibiting these signs may lack concentration, the ability to effectively absorb, learn or use information, and be poor at decision making. Cognitive symptoms often lead to emotional distress and make it hard for the person to earn a living, associate with people or lead a normal life.

All of the above could also be spirit interference.

If the medical profession was right about its diagnosis, then almost all mediums would be institutionalised or put on drugs. Any medium working with the spirit world will receive communication in one form or another. Some will hear voices, while others may see or get thoughts which aren't theirs. Many will feel the emotions or pains that the spirit was feeling at some time during its life.

According to the National Institute for Mental Health, 1% of the world's population has schizophrenia. That's 51 million people worldwide with the illness. In the United States, schizophrenia affects 7 in 1,000 people, so in a city with a population of 3 million that would be over 21,000 people at any given time. Has this got anything to do with people being more aware of the spirit world?

Although psychological disorders are widespread in a given population, only a small portion of those affected suffer from serious mental illness.

Schizophrenia is one of the psychological diseases diagnosed in the Diagnostic and Statistical Manual of Mental Disorders 4th edition (DSM-1V), and is categorised as an Axis 1 disorder. It is a "chronic, severe, and disabling brain disorder". The disorder affects 1% of the adult population in the world in a given year. Research shows that the probability of schizophrenia occurring is equal in both men and women and that the symptoms associated with the condition normally start showing between the ages of 16 and 30. Although it is very difficult to isolate symptoms of schizophrenia in teenagers, a combination of symptoms may make it possible to predict schizophrenia. Psychiatrists making a diagnosis of the disease may evaluate it by a thorough examination of the patient and their family members. Although no medical tests exist for schizophrenia, a number of factors may result in a higher probability of diagnosing the disease, although the factors may not confirm it. So does that mean that they can diagnose schizophrenia with or without 'a number of factors?' Much of the foregoing is guesswork: they can't even confirm it's a disease, let alone say what causes it.

Psychiatry is the new kid on the block and the profession is trying in all sorts of ways to justify itself, most of the time without a shred of evidence to back up its claims. Don't take my word for it: take a look at the following papers by Al Siebert PhD. and Laurence Stevens JD. There is a wealth of information and references for you to follow up if you want.

The Truth

This section is an edited version of an article written by Al Siebert, PhD that first appeared in the Journal of *Ethical Human Sciences and Services*. New York: Springer Publishing Company, Vol. 1, No. 2, Summer 1999, pp. 179-89 as "Brain Disease Hypothesis for Schizophrenia Disconfirmed by All Evidence." Available online at: www.SuccessfulSchizophrenia.org/articles/ehss.html

Reproduced with kind permission of Mrs Kristin Pintarich, Al Siebert's niece.

Prominent psychiatrists are stating that schizophrenia is a brain disease like Alzheimer's, Parkinson's or multiple sclerosis. These statements are disconfirmed by scientific facts: no neurologist can independently confirm the presence or absence of schizophrenia with laboratory tests, because the large majority of people diagnosed with schizophrenia, show no neuropathological or biochemical abnormalities, and some people without any symptoms of schizophrenia, have the same bio physiological abnormalities. People with schizophrenia do not usually progressively deteriorate, most improve over time. Psychotherapy and milieu therapy, (without medications), have led even the most severely disturbed individuals with schizophrenia to full recovery and beyond. Many people diagnosed with schizophrenia have recovered on their own without any treatment, something never accomplished by a person with Parkinson's, Alzheimer's or multiple sclerosis.

In July 1998 the chief of the Experimental Therapeutics Branch of the National Institute of Mental Health in the USA along with the director of the Mental Health Clinical Research Centre at the University of Iowa were interviewed on public radio. They are prominent psychiatric (experts), who stated, " things add up to produce a brain injury that we recognise as schizophrenia, it's just about universally recognised that it's a brain disease like all other brain diseases, Alzheimer's, Parkinson's Disease, multiple sclerosis and so on, there's no question this is a brain disorder".

These findings distort and misrepresent research findings published in the scientific literature in a number of different ways.

In 1902 Emil Kraeplin described Schizophrenia as not a "single disease". Fifty years later Eugen Bleuler agreed and described it as "The schizophrenias", professional references describe "the schizophrenias" as a group of conditions. The diversity of symptoms creates a major problem in the study of the disease and suggests schizophrenia is a group of diseases. In 1998 O'donnell and Grace say it is misleading to say schizophrenia is a single brain disease.

It was found in a study done in 1998 by Weikert & Weinberger that a few individuals diagnosed with schizophrenia show certain brain abnormalities, but the brain scans of the majority of people diagnosed with schizophrenia fall within normal ranges. Therefore the brain disease theory is weak. Some psychiatrists accredit unwarranted importance to weak evidence. For instance in a research study of childhood schizophrenia by (Nopoulos, Giedd, Andreason & Rapoport) in 1998 it was decided that patients with very early onset (childhood) forms of schizophrenia may have more severe developmental anomalies than those with adult onset. Out of 24 the data revealed only 3 showed abnormal enlargement of certain brain structures. 21 did not. In the healthy group, one subject had a similar brain anomaly.

It was found in a study by Ismail, Cantor-Grace & Mcneal in 1998 that schizophrenia patients displayed certain neurological abnormalities. Very similar abnormalities were found in their siblings even though they showed no clinical signs of schizophrenia. It was also found in a study by Andreason in 1995 that some people without symptoms of schizophrenia have brain abnormalities similar to those of schizophrenic subjects. Less than 35% of any given sample shows any brain abnormality in schizophrenia, the brains of the majority of patients diagnosed with schizophrenia are normal as far as researchers can tell, according to Lewine in 1998.Rarely do studies with positive findings take account of the effects of prolonged use of neuroleptics and other drugs.

Parkinson's, Alzheimer's and multiple sclerosis are brain diseases that progress towards life-long debilitation and are unpredictable for any one person, unlike schizophrenia, where there is solid evidence that people do recover, and it does not progress more after five years from its onset. The idea that the schizophrenias are essentially a progression towards dementia and death is a dreadful error. Almost a third of schizophrenics recover completely. These and other facts concerning the course and outcome of schizophrenia are certainly not typical of organic cerebral and metabolic disease. Studies of thousands of ex-patients in many countries show that only one-third of the individuals diagnosed as schizophrenic do not achieve full recovery or major improvement many years later.

One study showed in 1998 after a 15 year follow up that 77% had either full or partial remission. There have been many studies of ex-patients who were evaluated 20 to 35 years after discharge. Too many to list but the average recovery rate is 60-70%. Those who recovered include ex-patients once considered as the most severely disturbed. Courtney Harding and her colleagues (1987) evaluated 82 individuals who 20 to 25 years before, had been the most hopeless, chronically disturbed and backward patients when discharged from state hospital into a rehabilitation program. She emphasizes that "for one-half to two-thirds the long-term outcome was neither, downward or marginal, but an evolution to various degrees of productivity, social involvement, wellness and competent functioning" Many were found to be completely symptom free.

No brain disease has ever been cured with psychotherapy or the passage of time, but many therapists have reported observing with the use of psychotherapy and/or milieu therapy full recovery from schizophrenia. In the Soteria studies, young adults diagnosed as acutely schizophrenic were stabilised with no medication and non-professional helpers just as well, and quickly as a similar group sent to a psychiatric hospital. Many individuals diagnosed with schizophrenia have recovered on their own without medications or psychotherapy.

The best known case in recent times of spontaneous recovery from schizophrenia is that of John Forbes Nash. In 1949, at the age of 21 Nash wrote a Ph.D. thesis that established him as a mathematical genius. At the age of thirty he suffered a mental breakdown and was diagnosed with paranoid schizophrenia. Over the next twenty years he was hospitalised many times for brief periods. Then, for unknown reasons, Nash had a sudden remission. According to his ex-wife and sister, the two people who knew him best, his recovery was not due to any medication or psychological treatments.

There are those who have been diagnosed with schizophrenia who have progressed beyond recovery. Having a schizophrenic experience may have a beneficial effect in some cases on those who have been diagnosed, having a positive effect on their personality and psychological growth. According to John Weir Perry (1999) 85% of clients (all met DSM criteria forschizophrenia and were "severely psychotic") not only improved, without medication, but most went on growing after leaving.

There are those who experience a breakthrough to a higher level of mental and emotional performance after a schizophrenic episode. Siebert, (1996) and others stated that "with many patients who receive intensive and prolonged psychotherapy, we reach levels of integration and self-fulfilment that are far superior to those prevailing before the patient was psychotic" earlier Arieti (1974) wrote "some of my patients whom I consider cured have achieved important positions in life, in the academic world, as well as in other activities".

No one with Parkinson's, Alzheimer's, or multiple sclerosis is known to have fully recovered, and developed a level of health and functioning, superior to their pre-illness condition.

(The American Psychiatric Association 1994, Gottesman 1991) Stated the cause of schizophrenia is unknown. Andreasen stated during an interview that schizophrenia results from "multiple things, perhaps a genetic predisposition, nutritional factors early in life, viral infections, head injuries, exposure to toxin, exposure to drugs of various kinds, illicit drugs. All these things add up to produce a brain injury that we recognise as schizophrenia." This is a guess not a scientific fact. Why don't more people who are exposed to the forgoing risk factors, develop schizophrenia? Why is it that more individuals and siblings are not diagnosed with schizophrenia but have identical genetic predispositions, and are exposed to the same neurological trauma?

If the speculations made by Andreason were true, there would be more people with comparable "genetic predispositions," who would eventually develop schizophrenia from multiple neurological damage, caused by drinking and constant smoking, increasing environmental toxins, viral infections, poor nutrition, decreased immune system efficiency, an ageing brain and early stages of such brain diseases as Alzheimer's and Parkinson's. Proponents of the "brain disease" theory cannot explain why the schizophrenias occur so consistently in physically healthy young adults, aged 16-25, but rarely in anyone over forty, regardless of any psychological stressor.

There is no "worldwide" acknowledgement that schizophrenia is a brain disease "like all other brain diseases." Medical textbooks and pathology journals do not include schizophrenia as a pathophysiological condition (Schaler, 1998). Medical specialists that deal with neuropathology and neurological diseases such as Parkinson's and multiple sclerosis have nothing to say about the schizophrenias. None of the following neurology journals published articles on schizophrenia between1995-1998: Neurology (Official Journal of the American Academy of Neurology). The Neurological Sciences. Neuroradiology and Archives of Neurology. One article on the epidemiology of schizophrenia appeared in the Journal of Neurology, Neurosurgery and Psychiatry, but it had nothing to do with brain research. Most articles attempting to support the brain disease "theory" of schizophrenia appear in psychiatry and biopsychology journals

The idea that almost worldwide recognition of schizophrenia as a brain disease, is also disproved by statements from many psychiatrists and psychologists, clinically experienced with the schizophrenias, who see no convincing evidence for the theory.

Even the Diagnostic and Statistical Manual (fourth edition) of the American Psychiatric Association (1994) states plainly: "No laboratory findings have been identified that are diagnostic of schizophrenia" This statement highlights that the "brain disease" hypothesis stands or falls on simple criteria. A true brain disease must be identified and confirmed by laboratory tests. No blood chemistry, neurological, or brain scan test (or any other test) independently evaluated by a neurologist, biochemist, or pathologist who knows nothing about the patients clinical symptoms, is able to reliably discriminate between a person experiencing a first episode of schizophrenia and someone who is not. However such a test might well identify someone who has been taking neuroleptic medications for many years.

"Treatments" for schizophrenia are often worse than the

"disease." Pickar stated in his interview in (1998) that when people stop taking their medications "the consequences can be very severe." What Pickar did not report however, is that withdrawal symptoms can be disabling and mimic psychosis, and that long term drug use may be quite harmful. Neuroleptic medications may cause profound brain dysfunction and frequently lead to irreversible tardive dyskinesia in up to 50% of patients. This is a solidly established fact in psychiatry.

Many people diagnosed as schizophrenic say they are helped by neuroleptic drugs. It is professionally irresponsible, however, for Pickar and other schizophrenia psychiatrists not to inform the public that many people are seriously harmed by neuroleptic medications, and that many people can recover and maintain a full recovery from schizophrenia without medications.

Discussion by Al Siebert, Ph.D

Some psychiatrists drastically distort and misrepresent research findings published in the psychiatric literature. They constantly downplay evidence that most people with schizophrenia do not have brain or biochemical abnormalities, and that most people with similar abnormalities have no signs of schizophrenia. People with neuropathological diseases have never been cured by psychotherapy, nor found decades later to be fully recovered.

While some weak corwwrelations have been found between the presence of schizophrenic symptoms and certain brain abnormalities, a basic scientific principle remains: correlation does not mean causation. In some instances, an underlying cause may lead both to brain abnormalities and to schizophrenic symptoms. Some psychotherapists reporting cases of successful recovery from schizophrenia say that the symptoms can often be traced back to extremely traumatic childhood incidents that created powerful, conflicting feelings of loneliness and terror. What if some 'schizophrenic' conditions turn out to stem from some form of chronic childhood traumatic stress disorder that has had persistent effects on brain structure or function?

The real 'tragedy of schizophrenia' may be that thousands of people diagnosed with it are led to believe that they have a chronic, debilitating, progressive brain disease, like the incurable diseases of Alzheimer's, Parkinson's and multiple sclerosis. For many, this amounts to hearing themselves sentenced to a slow, painful, early death. Is this erroneous and misleading information contributing to the high suicide rates of people diagnosed as schizophrenic? Yet no-one ever dies of schizophrenia, even when untreated.

Responsible, scientifically accurate statements to the media about schizophrenia might be expressed as follows:

"A person diagnosed as having schizophrenia is expressing thoughts, feelings, and behaviours very disturbing to others and usually, but not necessarily, disturbing to the person expressing them. Research suggests that a few people diagnosed with schizophrenia have neurological complications, but many people with the same neurological profile do not develop schizophrenia. There is no known cure for schizophrenia because it isn't a disease and its cause is unknown. Some people benefit from medications that control their undesirable symptoms, some people are harmed by medications, and other people do better without medications. About one person in ten never recovers from the original disturbed or disturbing experience and the effects of repeated hospitalisations and drug use, but five or six out of ten can expect to fully recover or significantly improve. At present we cannot predict who will develop schizophrenia or why, who will recover or who will not. Further, we cannot explain why some people recover within weeks or months while others take from 5 to 20 years to recover."

There are currently 220,000 thousand people in the UK diagnosed with schizophrenia, according to the National Institute of Medical Health.

The Case Against Psychotherapy by Lawrence Stevens, J.D.

THE AUTHOR, Lawrence Stevens, is a lawyer whose practice has included representing psychiatric "patients". This work is not copyrighted. There are references to other papers at the back of this book in further reading.

"What we need are more kindly friends
and fewer professionals."
A statement by Jeffrey Masson, Ph.D.,
in his book *Against Therapy*
(Atheneum, 1988, p. XV)

The best person to talk with about your problems in life usually is a good friend. It has been said, "Therapists are expensive friends." Likewise, friends are inexpensive "therapists". Contrary to popular belief, and contrary to propaganda by mental health professionals, the training of psychiatrists, psychologists, and other mental health professionals does little or nothing to make them better equipped as counsellors or "therapists". It might seem logical for formal credentials like a Ph.D. in psychology or a psychiatrist's M.D. or D.O. degree or a social worker's M.S.W. degree to suggest a certain amount of competence on his or her part. The truth, however, is more often the opposite: In general, the less a person who is offering his or her services as a counsellor has in the way of formal credentials, the more likely he or she is to be a good counsellor, since such a counsellor has only competence (not credentials) to stand on. Generally, the best person for you to talk with is a person who has worked himself or herself through the same problems you face in the nitty-gritty of life. You usually will benefit if you avoid the "professionals" who claim their value comes from their years of academic study or professional training.

When I asked a licensed social worker with a Master of Social Work (M.S.W.) degree who shortly before had been employed in a psychiatric hospital whether she thought the psychiatrists she worked with had any special insight into people or their problems her answer was a resounding no. I asked the same question of a judge who had extensive experience with psychiatrists in his courtroom, and he gave me the same answer and made the point just as emphatically. Similarly, I sought an opinion from a high school teacher who worked as a counsellor helping young people overcome addiction or habituation to pleasure drugs who both as a teacher and as a drug counsellor had considerable experience with psychiatrists and people who consult them. I asked him if he felt psychiatrists have more understanding of human nature or human problems than himself or other people who are not mental health professionals. He thought a few moments and then replied, "No, as a matter of fact, I don't."

In his book *Against Therapy*, a critique of psychotherapy published in 1988, psychoanalyst Jeffrey Masson, Ph.D., speaks of what he calls "The myth of training" of psychotherapists. He says: "Therapists usually boast of their 'expertise,' the 'elaborate training' they have undergone. When discussing competence, one often hears phrases like 'he has been well trained,' or 'he has had specialized training.' People are rather vague about the nature of psychotherapy training, and therapists rarely encourage their patients to ask in any detail. They don't for a good reason: often their training is very modest. ... The most elaborate and lengthy training programs are the classic psychoanalytic ones, but this is not because of the amount of material that has to be covered. I spent eight years in my psychoanalytic training. In retrospect, I feel I could have learned the basic ideas in about eight hours of concentrated reading" (Athenaeum/Macmillan Co. p. 248).

Sometimes even psychiatrists and psychologists themselves will admit they have no particular expertise. Some of these admissions have come from people I have known as friends who happened to be practicing psychologists. Illustrative are the remarks of one Ph.D. psychologist who told me how amazed members of his family were that people would pay him $50 an hour just to discuss their problems with him. He admitted it really didn't make any sense, since they could do the same thing with lots of other people for free. "Of course," he said, "I'm still going to go to my office tomorrow and collect $50 an hour for talking with people." Due to inflation, today the cost is usually higher than $50 per hour.

In his book *The Reign of Error*, published in 1984, psychiatrist Lee Coleman, M.D., says "psychiatrists have no valid scientific tools or expertise" (Beacon Press, p. ix).

Garth Wood, M.D., a British psychiatrist, included the following statements in his book *The Myth of Neurosis* published in 1986: "Popularly it is believed that psychiatrists have the ability to 'see into our minds,' to understand the workings of the psyche, and possibly even to predict our future behaviour. In reality, of course, they possess no such skills. ... In truth there are very few illnesses in psychiatry, and even fewer successful treatments ... in the postulating of hypothetical psychological and biochemical causative processes, psychiatrists have tended to lay a smokescreen over the indubitable fact that in the real world it is not hard either to recognize or to treat the large majority of psychiatric illnesses. It would take the intelligent layman a long weekend to learn how to do it" (Harper & Row, 1986, p. 28-30; emphasis in original).

A cover article in *Time* magazine in 1979 titled "Psychiatry's Depression" made this observation: "Psychiatrists themselves acknowledge that their profession often smacks of modern alchemy - full of jargon, obfuscation and mystification, but precious little real knowledge" ("Psychiatry on the Couch", *Time* magazine, April 2, 1979, p. 74).

I once asked a social worker employed as a counsellor for troubled adolescents whose background included individual and family counselling if she felt the training and education she received as part of her M.S.W. degree made her more qualified to do her job than she would have been without it. She told me a part of her wanted to say yes, because after all, she had put a lot of time and effort into her education and training. She also mentioned a few minor benefits of having received the training. She concluded, however, "Most of the things I've done I think I could have done without the education."

Most mental health professionals however have an understandable emotional or mental block when it comes to admitting they have devoted, actually wasted, several years of their lives in graduate or professional education and are no more able to understand or help people than they were when they started. Many know it and won't, or will only rarely, admit it to others. Some cannot even admit it to themselves.

Hans J. Eysenck, Ph.D., is a psychology professor at the

University of London. In the December 1988 issue of *Psychology Today* magazine, the magazine's senior editor described Dr. Eysenck as "one of the world's best-known and most respected psychologists" (p. 27). This highly regarded psychologist states this conclusion about psychotherapy: "I have argued in the past and quoted numerous experiments in support of these arguments, that there is little evidence for the practical efficacy of psychotherapy...the evidence on which these views are based is quite strong and is growing in strength every year" ("Learning Theory and Behaviour Therapy", in *Behaviour Therapy and the Neuroses*, Pergamon Press, 1960, p. 4). Dr. Eysenck said that in 1960. In 1983 he said this: "The effectiveness of psychotherapy has always been the spectre at the wedding feast, where thousands of psychiatrists, psychoanalysts, clinical psychologists, social workers, and others celebrate the happy event and pay no heed to the need for evidence for the premature crystallization of their spurious orthodoxies" ("The Effectiveness of Psychotherapy: The Spectre at the Feast", *The Behavioural and Brain Sciences* 6, p. 290).

In *The Emperor's New Clothes: The Naked Truth About the New Psychology*, (Crossway Books, 1985) William Kirk Kilpatrick, a professor of educational psychology at Boston College, argues that we have attributed expertise to psychologists that they do not possess.

In 1983 three psychology professors at Wesleyan University in Connecticut published an article in The Behavioural and Brain Sciences, a professional journal, titled "An analysis of psychotherapy versus placebo studies". The abstract of the article ends with these words: "...there is no evidence that the benefits of psychotherapy are greater than those of placebo treatment" (Leslie Prioleau, et al., Vol. 6, p. 275).

George R. Bach, Ph.D., a psychologist, and co-author Ronald M. Deutsch, in their book *Pairing*, make this observation: "There are not enough therapists to listen even to a tiny fraction of these couples, and, besides, the therapy is not too successful. Popular impression to the contrary, when therapists, such as marriage counsellors, hold meetings, one primary topic almost invariably is: why is their therapy effective in only a minority of cases?" (Peter H. Wyden, Inc., 1970, p. 9; emphasis in original).

In his book *What's Wrong With the Mental Health Movement*, K. Edward Renner, Ph.D., a professor in the Department of Psychology at the University of Illinois at Urbana, makes this observation in his chapter titled "Psychotherapy": "When control groups are included, those patients recover to the same extent as those patients receiving treatment. The enthusiastic belief expressed by therapists about their effectiveness, in spite of the negative results, illustrates the problem of the therapist who must make important human decisions many times each day. He is in a very awkward position unless he believes in what he is doing" (Nelson-Hall Publishers, 1975, pp. 138-139; emphasis in original).

An example of this occurred at the psychiatric clinic at the Kaiser Foundation Hospital in Oakland, California. Of 150 persons who sought psychotherapy, all were placed in psychotherapy except for 23 who were placed on a waiting list. After six months, doctors checked on those placed on the waiting list to see how much better the people receiving psychotherapy were doing than those receiving none. Instead, the authors of the study found that "The therapy patients did not improve significantly more than did the waiting list controls" (Martin L. Gross, The Psychological Society, Random House, 1978, p. 18).

In the second edition of his book *Is Alcoholism Hereditary?* published in 1988, Donald W. Goodwin, M.D., says "There is hardly any scientific evidence that psychotherapy for alcoholism or any other condition helps anyone" (Ballantine Books, 1988, p. 180).

British psychiatrist Garth Wood, M.D., criticizes modern day "psychotherapy" in his book *The Myth of Neurosis* published in 1986 with these words: "These misguided myth-makers have encouraged us to believe that the infinite mysteries of the mind are as amenable to their professed expertise as plumbing or an automobile engine. This is rubbish. In fact these talk therapists, practitioners of cosmetic psychiatry, have no relevant training or skills in the art of living life. It is remarkable that they have fooled us for so long. ... Cowed by their status as men of science, deferring to their academic titles, bewitched by the initials after their names, we, the gullible, lap up their pretentious nonsense as if it were the gospel truth. We must learn to recognize them for what they are - possessors of no special knowledge of the human psyche, who have, nonetheless, chosen to earn their living from the dissemination of the myth that they do indeed know how the mind works" (pp. 2-3).

The superiority of conversation with friends over professional psychotherapy is illustrated in the remarks of a woman interviewed by Barbara Gordon in a book published in 1988: "For Francesca, psychotherapy was a mixed blessing." It helps, but not nearly as much as a few intense, good friends,' she said. '...I pay a therapist to listen to me, and at the end of forty-five minutes he says, 'That's all the time we have; we'll continue next week.' A friend, on the other hand, you can call any hour and say, 'I need to talk to you.' They're there, and they really love you and want to help." In an interview with another woman on the same page of the same book, Ms' Gordon was told this, referring to pain from losing a husband: "Good shrinks can probably deal with it; the two I went to didn't help" (Barbara Gordon, *Jennifer Fever*, Harper & Row, 1988, p. 132).

The June 1986 issue of *Science 86* magazine included an article by Bernie Zilbergeld, a psychologist, suggesting that "we're hooked on therapy when talking to a friend might do as well." He cited a Vanderbilt University study that compared professional "psychotherapy" with discussing one's problems with interested but untrained persons: "Young men with garden variety neuroses were assigned to one of two groups of therapists. The first consisted of the best professional psychotherapists in the area, with an average 23 years of experience; the second group was made up of college professors with reputations of being good people to talk to but with no training in psychotherapy. Therapists and professors saw their clients for no more than 25 hours. The results: "Patients undergoing psychotherapy with college professors showed ... quantitatively as much improvement as patients treated by experienced professional psychotherapists" (p. 48). Zilbergeld pointed out that "the Vanderbilt study mentioned earlier is far from the only one debunking the claims of professional superiority" (ibid, p. 50).

Martin L. Gross, a member of the faculty of The New School For Social Research and an Adjunct Assistant Professor of Social History at New York University, has argued that "the concept that a man who is trained in medicine or a Ph.D. in psychology has a special insight into human nature is false" (quoted in "And ACLU Chimes In: Psychiatric Treatment May Be Valueless", *Behaviour Today*, June 12, 1978, p. 3).

Implicit in the idea of "psychotherapy" is the belief that "psychotherapists" have special skills and special knowledge that are not possessed by other people. In making this argument against "psychotherapy", I am arguing only that conversation with psychotherapists is no better than conversation with other people. In his defence of psychotherapy in a book published in 1986, psychiatrist E. Fuller Torrey makes this argument: "Saying that psychotherapy does not work is like saying that prostitution does not work; those enjoying the benefits of these personal transactions will continue doing so, regardless of what the experts and researchers have to say" (*Witchdoctors and Psychiatrists: The Common Roots of Psychotherapy and Its Future*, Jason Aronson, Inc., p. 198). If you really are desperate for someone to talk to, then "psychotherapy" may in fact be enjoyable. However, if you have a good network of friends or family who will talk to you confidentially and with your best interests at heart, there is no need for "psychotherapy". Just as a happily married man or a man with a good sexually intimate relationship with a steady girlfriend is unlikely to have reason to hire a prostitute, people with good friendships with other people are unlikely to need "psychotherapy".

What if you need information about how to solve a problem your family and friends can't help you with? In that case usually the best person for you to talk to is someone who has lived through or is living through the same problem you face. Sometimes a good way to find such people is attending meetings of a group organized to deal with the kind of problem you have. Examples (alphabetically) are Alcoholics Anonymous, Alzheimer's Support groups, Agoraphobia Self-Help groups, Al-Anon (for relatives of alcoholics), Amputee Support groups, Anorexia/Bulimia support groups, The Aphasia Group, Arthritics Caring Together, Children of Alcoholics, Coping With Cancer, Debtors Anonymous, divorce adjustment groups, father's rights associations (for divorced men), Gamblers Anonymous, herpes support and social groups such as HELP, Mothers Without Custody, Nar-Anon (for relatives of narcotics abusers), Narcotics Anonymous, Overeaters Anonymous, Parents Anonymous, Parents in Shared Custodies, Parents Without Partners, Potsmokers Anonymous, Resolve, Inc., (a support group that deals with the problems of infertility and miscarriage), Shopaholics Ltd., singles groups, Smokers Anonymous, The Stuttering Support Group, women's groups, and unwed mothers assistance organizations. Local newspapers often have listings of meetings of such organizations. Someone who is a comrade with problems similar to yours and who has accordingly spent much of his or her life trying to find solutions for those problems is far more likely to know the best way for you to deal with your situation than a "professional" who supposedly is an expert at solving all kinds of problems for all kinds of people. The myth of professional psychotherapy training and skill is so widespread, however, that you may find people you meet in self-help groups will recommend or refer you to a particular psychiatrist, psychologist, or social worker. If you hear this, remember what you read (above) in this pamphlet and disregard these recommendations and referrals and get whatever counselling you need from nonprofessional people in the group who have direct experience in their own lives with the kind of problem that troubles you. You will probably get better advice and - importantly - you will avoid psychiatric stigma.

In their book *A New Guide To Rational Living*, Albert Ellis, Ph.D., a New York City psychologist, and Robert A. Harper, Ph.D., say they follow "an educational rather than a psychodynamic or a medical model of psychotherapy" (Wilshire Book Co., 1975, p. 219). In his book *Get Ready, Get Set...Prepare to Make Psychotherapy A Successful Experience For You*, psychotherapist and psychology professor Harvey L. Saxton, Ph.D., writes: "What is psychotherapy? Psychotherapy is simply a matter of re-education. Re-education implies letting go of the outmoded and learning the new and workable. Patients, in one sense, are like students; they need the capacity and willingness to engage in the process of relearning" (University Press of America, 1993, p. 1). In their book *When Talk Is Not Cheap, Or How To Find the Right Therapist When You Don't Know Where To Begin,* psychotherapist Mandy Aftel, M.A., and Professor Robin Lakoff, Ph.D., say "Therapy...is a form of education" (Warner Books, 1985, p. 29). Since so-called psychotherapy is a form of education, not therapy, you need not a doctor or therapist but a person who is qualified to educate in the area of living in which you are having difficulty. The place to look for someone to talk to is where you are likely to find someone who has this knowledge. Someone whose claim to expertise is a "professional" psychotherapy training program rarely if ever is the person who can best advise you.

Observations

In many of the houses I have visited, there has been some sort of traumatic occurrence such as a death in the family or the loss of a baby, or some other emotional stress or from which we have been able to track the first episode of disturbance. This happens because the individual's emotions have been heightened by the event, and they have become more sensitive to their surroundings. When this happens, they can be influenced by the spirit world. In almost every case we have been successful in resolving the issues that have presented themselves, partly by explanations and by talking to and helping the lost or misguided spirits on their journey. There is no time in spirit: it is always 'now', and this can lead to the spirits being confused when they find out how long they have been lost. Humanity lives by the clock, otherwise nobody would be where they wanted or needed to be at the right moment. We have ordered our days according to night and day and to the seasons of the year. This is unnecessary in the spirit world as they don't eat, sleep or age and everyone is just a thought away.

Spirit can be lost for as long as it takes for them to realise what has happened and where they are. If they are aware of what's happened, but don't believe in an afterlife, then they will stay in their thought pattern until they are encouraged out of it by their loved ones or guides. It can take five minutes or it can take many years: it depends on the individual circumstances and the spirit's understanding.

Many of the people we meet who are having spiritual problems end up at spiritualist churches, after having exhausted all other avenues of inquiry which have been examined and found inadequate. It stands to reason that if they are hearing voices and they are not mad, then who else but mediums might understand what is happening and be able to help? Mediums and mystics have been helping lost souls for hundreds of years to find their way home.

Case 1

The following is about a woman called Sonia who had been diagnosed as a paranoid schizophrenic.

I met Sonia at a spiritualist church where I was working. Sonia told me she was experiencing major problems in all parts of her life and asked if I could help her. I asked her to tell me about herself and what was going on.

Sonia is a professional businesswoman who has been running her own business for the past five years: she employs three people. She is aged about 45, tall and comfortably dressed. She lives alone after splitting up with her long-term partner eight years ago. She likes to keep fit and used to go jogging with a group three times a week, but that's all stopped now as she is fearful of going out. Sonia said she was seeing a counsellor once a week about depression and had been referred to a psychiatrist. The psychiatrist had diagnosed her as paranoid schizophrenic and prescribed Prozac in the first instance to try and calm her down.

I asked her to tell me what she was experiencing.

Sonia told me she wasn't sleeping and had big mood changes. She felt she was being watched all the time and had become very hesitant about leaving the house. She said it felt like she was being sexually assaulted and as she lived on her own, this was very disturbing. I sensed there were a number of negative spirits around her, playing with her moods and temperament. She said she would get angry for no reason and had trouble holding a conversation with people, as she couldn't find the words to say. She always had the feeling people were looking down on her, and putting her down. Within ten minutes her demeanour would change and she would become hyper and couldn't stop talking. It was as if she were a different person.

She said that although she had been diagnosed as paranoid schizophrenic, she didn't accept the diagnosis. She said she had been to a few open circles at the spiritualist church, and knew she could hear spirit and wasn't mentally ill. The spirits were interfering with her daily life and giving her emotions that she knew weren't hers. Could I help her to control what was going on? From my experience it was clear she was being attacked by discarnate spirits. I spoke to her about what was happening and assured her she wasn't mad, and if she would let me, I would help her remove her troublesome spirits. She was wary, so I suggested she talk to a few people at the church to reassure her that I was genuine. It was fortunate that one of the mediums there had experienced similar problems which I had resolved for her about a year earlier. After talking to that medium, she came and said if I could help it would be much appreciated. I told her we would put protection around her house, so the spirits that were there couldn't get out, and no others could get in. I explained that it might get a bit more active, or it might go very quiet - you could never tell. We would come and remove everything inside the protection, and - once it was clear - the protection would remain, so no more could get in. I spoke to my team members and we arranged an evening that was mutually convenient.

When I telephoned her to confirm the time and date, I asked when it had all started. This is what she said:

"About three years ago my brother committed suicide and I couldn't stop crying. I went to the doctor and he put me on antidepressants but things got worse. I was lethargic and couldn't concentrate. Gradually I settled down and started to wean myself off the antidepressants with the doctor's blessing, but things got worse so I continued taking them. As I started to get back to normal, I was aware something wasn't right - I started getting mood changes and things were happening that I couldn't explain. Things were being moved and I was hearing noises when there was no-one there. Thinking about it now, it was a gradual process. Only by looking back can I see how things changed. At first I would just be depressed for no apparent reason; I seem to remember getting headaches a lot and sometimes my whole body ached. I started having dreams, which after a while turned into nightmares and I would wake up in a cold sweat. That was when I was lucky enough to get to sleep. Sometimes I would be very tired, but when I went to bed I would feel wide awake, until in the end I would fall into a troubled sleep. I used to get up full of energy but now I have trouble getting out of bed - I don't feel as though I've had much sleep at all. I wake up in the middle of the night thinking I heard something and have trouble getting back to sleep. Sometimes it feels as though someone's standing by the bed watching me."

"Okay," I said. "We'll see if we can sort it out for you - call me in the meantime if you have any problems and we'll see you in a couple of days."

As we walked into her house it was like walking into a solid wall of negativity. We could all feel the misery and fear that pervaded the whole house. The house was freezing even though the radiators were hot. As we walked along the hallway it felt like we were walking into a very dark place. Sonia looked very frightened and worn out. She said:

"I'm so tired I can't think straight. I'd forgotten you were coming. Please make yourselves comfortable - would you like a cup of tea?"

"In a little while," I said. "First we need to settle you down and take away your headache and help you to feel more at ease."

I sat her on a chair and asked her if it was okay for Vanessa to give her some healing for her headache, which she agreed to. After it had subsided she asked:

"How did you do that? I've taken pills and tried to sleep but I couldn't shift it."

"I asked my guides to block the interference you were getting from the discarnate spirit who was giving you the pain - we'll talk to him soon. I just wanted you to feel more comfortable," said Vanessa.

"Do you mean spirit can do that? Why would they?"

"By causing you pain, it drains your energy and affects all parts of your life, which makes it easier to control you. When they get into your aura you will feel the pain as if it's your own. Some don't know you can feel it, but others do it on purpose to wear you down."

We sat down and I asked Sonia:

"Would you like to tell us what's been going on over the past week?"

"Since I spoke to you it's been a lot worse," she said. "I've had banging noises and people talking, and last night I woke up with someone in bed with me. When I screamed it went but I couldn't go back to bed. I've had aches and pains all week - as soon as one pain goes, I get another somewhere else. I had to take three days off work. I felt so insecure and had no confidence in myself or my ability to do my job. In fact if I'd remembered you were coming I would've phoned you and asked you not to come because I was so down. I've still got this feeling of someone watching me and I haven't been out since Wednesday."

"I did say it might get worse," I said. "If you'd phoned I could've calmed things down for you. Never mind, we're here now so we'll sort things out."

"I didn't realise it wasn't me - my counsellor said I was very depressed and needed something for my nerves."

"Have you told your counsellor about hearing voices and being molested?"

"No, I thought if I told her that she would section me."

"Why did you think I would believe you?"

"Because when I was speaking to that medium at the church, she told me she'd been molested and you'd stopped it happening to her, so I hoped you could help me too. As for hearing voices, I knew you would believe me because you understand that part of it since you hear voices yourself."

"Okay, are you hearing voices now?"

"Yes there's a lot of chatter and arguments going on; it's as though I'm in a room full of people all talking at once. It's gone quiet now and someone is talking to me, telling me I'm useless, and why bother talking to you about it because you won't believe me."

"Yes and they're also telling you to get rid of us as we won't be able to help, aren't they?"

"Yes they are, so I'm not crazy - can you stop it?"

"We're certainly going to try. Let me explain what we're going to do and then we'll get started, alright?"

I told Sonia how we were going to work.

"Danny, Vanessa and I all work differently but complement each other. Danny is a trance medium and the spirits will come through him so that you can hear what they have to say. Vanessa, who is a healer, is aware of the spirits that are in the house - she also backs me up by talking to those who are afraid of men. I'm able to pick up on the spirits also and - with the help of my guides - control the proceedings. If at any time you feel uncomfortable or in pain please tell me, as I will be focussing on the spirit and

I need to know if you get attacked. I'm not saying you will, but sometimes they will attack the most vulnerable to distract us."

Once Sonia was settled I asked Vanessa what she was aware of.

"I have a man who is about thirty-five - he's making me feel sick."

"Okay, Danny, can you get him?"

"Yes I've been watching him," said Danny. "I'll bring him through."

"Okay, you can stop that now - you've got our attention," I said.

"Good. Now you know what I can do - you'd better leave or I'll have to show you what else I can do," said the spirit, through Danny.

"Why are you doing that to people? It's not very nice"

"I can do a lot worse."

"Not any more you can't - we're going to restrict you so you'll behave yourself while we're talking."

"What have you done? I can't move!"

"No but you can still talk - why are you doing this?"

"Because I can and I like a bit of sex."

"Well you can't bother the women any more. What's your name?"

"Mind your own business. I can do what I like - you can't stop me."

"We will if we have to, but I'd rather you stopped yourself."

"Why would I want to do that? I've got her in the house all to myself. I'm going to make the most of it."

"I take it you know what's happened to you?"

"Of course I do - that's what makes it better. They can't stop me, now and I can do whatever I like. Women, they think they're so high and mighty, well now it's time for them to find out they're not."

"We can and will stop you from preying on innocent women. They've done nothing to you."

"No women's innocent - look how they lead you on and then take you for all you've got and dump you."

"That may be your experience, but not all women are the same. Would you like to go to heaven?"

"No I'm quite happy here thanks."

"In that case we'll have to remove you and stop you from interfering with people. We're going to put you in a bubble of calming energy: when you decide to go to heaven you just have to ask. If, on the other hand, you don't want to go to heaven then you can wait for your family. In the meantime you won't be able to bother anyone else. Goodbye."

Danny came back and said:

"He was surrounded by our guides and marched off the premises. They were talking to him, trying to make him see the error of his ways, but he was just swearing at them, so they left him in the bubble of light to calm down."

"Okay. How do you feel, Vanessa?"

"I'm okay," she said. "I just blocked him until Danny had him."

"Is that the one who was in bed with me? He's horrible." Sonia said.

"We won't be seeing him again," I said. "Now let's see what else you've got here. I'm aware of two men standing behind you. Danny, they're not very nice and keep changing how they look. One looks like a gargoyle and keeps pulling horrible faces. Can you bring him through so we can have a little chat?"

"I see lots of faces when I'm trying to sleep," said Sonia

"It's not uncommon - they're just trying to scare you. Take no notice. Can you bring him through please, Danny?"

When he came through it was obvious he was trying to get away, but once Danny had him he must have realised he couldn't, because he stopped struggling.

"Hello, it's a waste of time fighting - you can't go anywhere until we let you, so settle down. You never know - you might gain something," I said.

"You've got nothing I want and I'll soon sort him out - then I'll be after you."

"Why are you so aggressive? What're your intentions towards this lady?"

"That's none of your business. What're you going to do, get your bible out and start reading prayers? Go on."

"We don't need to say prayers - we both know they will have no effect. Now it's just a question of whether you want help or not."

"How do you think you can help me?"

"We could take you to heaven so that you could be with your family and friends."

"I don't want to go to heaven - I'm having too much fun here, so I'm staying."

"Sorry you feel that way. There's nothing left to say except you'll be removed from here and placed in a bubble of calming energy. That way you can't interfere with anyone else, and you will have time to reconsider your position. When you decide you want to be with your family you only have to ask. Goodbye."

Danny's face got angry and it was clear he was having a struggle; then it cleared and he opened his eyes.

"He was a nasty so and so," he said. "As soon as you said goodbye he went berserk - he tried to attack me by making me feel ill and giving me all sorts of pains. It felt a bit weird; first I felt like I wanted to be sick and had a cold sweat, then I had pains all over my body at once. I asked my guide to remove him and it all went along with him. I watched him being taken away - he was fighting all the time."

"Are you okay now?" I asked.

"Yes I feel fine - it only lasted a couple of seconds."

He was reluctant to go, but he was with our guides who would try to help him.

Sonia started fidgeting and her face went red and she said:

"There's someone touching my shoulder."

I was aware of a lady beside Sonia.

"Okay we'll get her now. Danny, would you mind?"

Danny brought through the woman who was touching Sonia as she started to swear. I was aware of three other women who were also with her.

"Go away, you nosy so-and-so - who do you think you are?" Not quite the words she used.

"Would you restrict her so she can't talk, for a minute please?" I asked. Then I asked, "Sonia, are you okay now?"

"Yes, it suddenly went," said Sonia.

I addressed the spirit woman: "Now you can stop swearing and calm down. You're not going anywhere until we've spoken. You can let her speak now, Danny."

"You have no right to interfere," she said. "It's taken me ages to set this place up."

"We have every right - we've been invited, which is more than I can say for you. Why are you causing so much trouble? It's not necessary. Do you know what's happened to you?"

"Of course I know and I can do what I like."

"Not here you can't. If you're going to carry on with what you're doing we'll have to remove you."

"I've spent too much time setting this place up. I'm not going to stop now. I'm just starting to enjoy myself."

"Don't you think you would feel better if you were with your family? You could enjoy yourself without upsetting other people and you would be safe - you wouldn't have to prove how tough you are."

"I'm not going anywhere. I've just told you."

"We're offering to take you to heaven where you can have a bit of peace and be with David. Are you sure?" Whilst talking to the entranced spirit, I am also in communication with my guides who supply relevant information as I need it. This helps when it is someone they have known, sometimes to encourage the entranced spirit to leave and find peace with someone they trust.

"Yes I'm sure - now bugger off."

"I'm sorry you feel that way. We'll have to remove you from here and restrict your freedom while our guides have a long chat with you. Maybe they can help you. They're going to take your three friends too and have a chat with them. You can go with them now good bye."

When Danny came back, Sonia said:

"She was really nasty - she's been doing things to me for ages. I didn't know how to stop it."

"She's gone now so you won't be bothered by her anymore," I said.

Vanessa said. "There's a woman sitting on the arm of the chair watching - she looks like she's in pain."

"I'll bring her through," said Danny.

"Hello - it's alright, you're safe now. Would you like to tell me your name?" Vanessa said.

"I'm Joan. Who are you?"

"We've come to help you. I can see you're in a lot of pain - let's take that away for you. There - is that better?"

"Yes that's wonderful - how did you do that?"

"We just gave you healing. Now do you know what's happened to you?"

"Yes I died - I jumped off a cliff."

"I see, when was that?"

"When I was twenty two in 1935."

"I see and where do people go when they die?"

"They go to heaven, but I took my own life so they won't let me in - I've committed a sin."

"That's not true. We can take you to heaven if you'd like. You can go and be with Edward. Would you like that?"

"Yes I would, but I think I've been making that woman feel my pain. Each time I went and tried to talk to her, she started holding her back and rubbing her arms and legs. When I moved away she seemed to be alright."

"Well we know you didn't do it on purpose - you were just trying to get help. Can you open your eyes and tell me what you can see?"

"I can see a big light - it's like looking down a tunnel. Is that heaven?"

"Yes. If you walk forward, you'll see Edward waiting for you."

"Oh yes I can see him now - can I go to him?"

"Yes. Be happy; you'll be safe now."

While Vanessa was talking to the woman, she noticed a small boy standing in the corner watching her. He didn't look well - he had blood running down his face and his arm was broken - so we decided to see if we could help him. I asked Danny if he could tune in to him and bring him through gently.

"Hello, you're Adrian aren't you?" I said and waited. I wasn't going to rush him because he looked very frightened.

"Yes, hello," he said. "Why can't I find my mummy? She was here just now."

"We'll find your mummy for you in a minute, but first we need to help you feel safe and comfortable," I said.

"Who are you? Mummy said I mustn't talk to strangers unless she or daddy are there."

"I'm called Mike and this is Vanessa - we're here to help you. Are you in any pain?"

"No I'm cold and lost and my arm hurts. Can I talk to the

lady please?"

"Hello," said Vanessa. "Let's make you better and warm and then we'll see if we can help you. Is that better?"

"Yes thank you."

"Good - now do you know what's happened to you?"

"I'm in this horrible house. I was on holiday with mummy and daddy and then I got very cold and it all went black and when I opened my eyes I was here. Where is this house?"

"This house belongs to the lady sitting over there. What's the last thing you remember, before you found yourself here?"

"We were on holiday and mummy said we could go swimming in the river. I was just paddling by the side when fell in and went under the water. I couldn't breathe. I don't remember anything after that, until I was here."

"Can you swim?"

"No, well a little bit."

"Well you fell in a hole under the water and you got taken out into the river by the current. What do you think must have happened to you?"

"If I was under water I must be dead - you can't breathe under water."

"Yes, that's right. Do you know what year it was?" I asked.

"Yes I just had my birthday I'm 8 so it was 1956."

"That was a long time ago. Where do people go when they die?"

"Mummy says if you're good you go to heaven. Why didn't I go? I haven't been bad."

"No you haven't, but because it was so sudden that you didn't know you had died. You were looking for your mummy in the wrong place. Your mummy and sister are in heaven. Would you like us to take you there?"

"Yes please - is daddy there too?"

"No he's not there yet, but your granddad is and lots of other people you know."

"Where's daddy then? Has he got lost too? Can you find him?"

"Your daddy is still alive. Mummy will take you to see him once you've settled down. Now shall we go and find mummy?"

"Yes please, I miss her and my sister and daddy."

"I know you do. Open your eyes really wide and tell me what

you can see."

"I can see a big tunnel and there's a big light in it."

"That's the way to heaven where your mummy is. There are a lot of other children trying to find their mummy too. Will you help me to take them to heaven as well?"

"Yes okay - can we go now?"

"In a moment. Let's get all the children together - we don't want to lose anyone, do we? Right, now we can go into the tunnel. Here, hold my hand - off we go. What can you see now?"

"I can see mummy and my sister. How did they get here?"

"They have been in heaven for a while. Would you like to go and stay with them? Your granddad is there too -can you see him?"

"Yes - thank you for helping us all. Bye."

With that, he went skipping off to heaven and Danny - after making sure he got there safely - opened his eyes.

"There's an elderly man standing next to me. Danny, are you aware of him? He's about 70 and he's wearing a flat cap and glasses." I said.

"Yes he's about 5ft 5in and a little bit tubby - is that him?" asked Danny.

"Yes - would you ask him to come and talk to us, please?"

The man came through and said:

"Can you hear me? I need help. I don't seem to be able to talk to people - they just ignore me?"

"Yes, we can hear you. How can we help?" I said.

"I woke up this morning and my wife was crying. When I asked her what was wrong, she just ignored me and went downstairs. I followed her down asking what was wrong, but she didn't reply. She went to the telephone and spoke to the doctor."

"Do you know what she said?"

"She said could they come quickly as she thought I had died."

"How did you feel when she said that?"

"I told her I was fine - if only she would look at me, she would see."

"Had it occurred to you that perhaps you had died and now are spirit and she couldn't see you?"

"No, I felt the same. Have I died?"

"Yes I'm afraid so. What year was it?"

46

"It's 1967 - it was only this morning."

"Unfortunately it's now 2012. You've been gone for 56 years now. Where do people go when they die?"

"That's a long time - it just feels like this morning. Don't they go to heaven or somewhere like that?"

"Yes and if you like we'll take you to see your wife and family."

"I think it's about time I went. I expect she'll give me an earful for getting lost. Oh well, it'll be worth it to see her again."

"Okay, open your eyes and tell me what you can see."

"I can see a bright light, it's like a tunnel."

"That's the way to heaven. Shall we go?"

"Yes please. I'm glad I met you. Oh there she is - can I go to her?"

"Yes be happy, goodbye."

"Goodbye and thank you."

We then removed a lot more people who were lost, both adults and children, until there was no-one left and the house was clear. We were there for four hours: sometimes it takes more than one visit. It depends mostly on the person who is experiencing the problem. I explained to Sonia about how to keep safe and we answered her questions over a cup of tea. Vanessa told Sonia about healing and asked if she would like some. Sonia said yes and they arranged a day when they were both free.

We saw Sonia a couple of weeks later and it was clear that things were better. She was smiling and didn't look worried anymore. She asked:

"Should I continue taking the pills the doctor gave me? I don't feel depressed anymore."

Vanessa said: "I think you should see how it goes. If, in a couple of weeks, you're feeling okay then go and see the doctor and see what they say."

Over the next month we kept in contact with her and she was a different person. She had come for healing a few times and Vanessa said she was a lot calmer now. Sonia was confident and happy, no aches or pains and more relaxed. She was sleeping better and felt much more alive in the mornings. She did see the doctor and told her she didn't think she needed the pills anymore. The doctor said to cut down over the following few weeks and see how she was.

She now comes to the church regularly and is a changed

person. It's six months since we visited her and she has gone from strength to strength. She helps out at the church and hopes to join a circle so she can learn to help other people who are suffering the way she had been.

This type of spirit interference relates to symptoms similar to paranoid schizophrenia and schizoaffective disorder - both very troubling, but not an illness of the brain.

Types of Personality Disorder

Multiple Personality Disorder (MPD), it is suggested, is a mental disorder characterised by at least two distinct identities or dissociated personality states. They alternately control a person's behaviour, and are accompanied by memory loss of important information that is not explained by ordinary forgetfulness. These symptoms are not accounted for by substance abuse, seizures, other medical conditions, or imaginative play in children. Diagnosis is often difficult as they overlap, or are similar to, other mental disorders.

The foregoing paragraph clearly explains possession: if there is no medical explanation, then surely the spirit world should be considered as a possibility. Some of those in spirit are able to take control of people who, for whatever reason, have low self-esteem and to control their thoughts and feelings. When you get two or more spirits controlling someone, each spirit has their own thought process and memories. Therefore when the person does something while controlled by one spirit, they won't necessarily log that action in their mind. If this happens under different spirit controls, their memory of events will be disjointed.

The medical profession states that diagnosis is often difficult as there are symptoms similar to other mental disorders.

There are a number of medical conditions that can cause psychosis: here are nine examples:

-Disorders causing delirium (toxic psychosis) in which consciousness is disturbed.

-Neurodevelopmental disorders and chromosomal abnormalities.

-Neurodegenerative disorders, such as Alzheimer's disease, dementia with Lewy bodies and Parkinson's disease.

-Focal neurological disease, such as stroke, brain tumours, multiple sclerosis and some forms of epilepsy.

-Malignancy (typically via masses in the brain, para-neoplastic syndromes, or drugs used to treat cancer)

-Infectious and post-infectious syndromes, including infections causing delirium, viral encephalitis, HIV, malaria, Lyme disease, and syphilis.

-Endocrine disease, thyroid problems. Sex hormownes can also affect psychotic symptoms and sometimes childbirth can provoke psychosis, termed puerperal psychosis.

-Inborn errors of metabolism, porphyria and metachromatic leukodystrophy.

-Nutritional deficiency such as vitamin B12 deficiency.

This list is not exhaustive but it can be seen that, although diagnosis can be difficult, once these complaints have been tested for and eliminated then there can be only one cause to consider, which is not organic.

They are looking for problems with the brain, which is just an organ of the body. It would be well worth considering the mind being separate from the brain, and that it can be influenced by discarnate spirits.

Dissociative identity disorder (DID) and MPD are just two names for the same thing. It is, they say, one of the most controversial psychiatric disorders, with no clear agreement regarding its diagnosis or treatment, which is not really surprising if they don't consider outside influences like spirit.

When a medium goes into trance, the spirits that come through have their own memories and personalities, which are distinct from that of the medium. They also have their own way of talking. Their phraseology is totally different from the way the medium would speak ordinarily, and their knowledge will also be from the spirit's perspective, not the medium's. There are those in spirit who are bored, disgruntled or just plain nasty, who didn't want to die and sometimes don't even know they have died. Some spirits want to continue to live in this world and do so by taking over people's minds - they don't or won't move on of their own accord. Then there are those who like to control others; this they can do through the mind. It's not a big step to understand this, as there are plenty of drugs that humanity uses and the most obvious and oldest way of controlling someone's mind is through hypnosis or drugs.

When a person is hypnotised, their state of mind is almost the same as when trance takes place. In the period 1850-1930s, most mediums who went into trance had a mesmeriser to assist them to get into a receptive state for spirit to come through.

DID symptoms range from common lapses in attention, becoming distracted by something else, and daydreaming, to pathological dissociative disorders.

When a medium is working, communicating with discarnate spirits, their attention is not on their surroundings. It is on the communicator who is talking to them from the world of spirit. Imagine someone who doesn't know they can communicate with spirit. They would have lapses in concentration and would also be distracted, or appear to be daydreaming. It's a common misconception that all mediums hear voices - many just get thoughts or feelings. How would someone who has not been trained, recognise what's happening to them? There are, of course, people who do have mental problems, but to diagnose their particular problem without considering the spirit world is like working with only half the information. (Source) Wikipedia.

It's thought that DID rarely resolves spontaneously and symptoms are said to vary over time. The prognosis is poor, especially for those with underlying problems that may stem from a genuine mental disorder. At the moment there is not enough understanding of the brain, let alone the mind. The prevalence of DID increased greatly in the latter half of the twentieth century, along with the number of identities (often referred to as 'alters') claimed by patients. It is three to nine times more common in females than in males. It has been suggested that DID may also be a product of techniques employed by some therapists, especially those using hypnosis. DID became a popular diagnosis in the 1970s, 80s and 90s but it is unclear if the actual incident of the disorder increased, or was more recognised by clinicians, or if socio-cultural factors caused an increase in presentations. The unusual number of diagnoses after 1980, clustered around a small number of clinicians and the suggestibility characteristic of those with DID, support the hypothesis that DID is therapist-induced. The unusual clustering of diagnoses has also been explained as due to lack of training among clinicians to recognise cases of DID.

It's well known that women are more sensitive to the spirit world than men, so not surprising they're more susceptible to spirit influence than males. The fact that hypnosis has been more widely used since the 1970s indicates spirit are using the hypnotic state as a way into the consciousness of patients. This is understandable when you consider the hypnotic state is almost the same as the trance state, and clinicians don't understand the mind, or how it interacts with the conscious state of the patient. The very fact that diagnoses were originally clustered around a small area, and the inability to understand the conscious and subconscious mind, suggests the clinicians haven't grasped the distinction between brain and mind. Over the past 50 years, more people have gained a greater awareness of the spirit world, especially with the wide media coverage, and the fact that mediumship was hidden behind closed doors until recently. In 1951 the witchcraft act in Britain was repealed and mediums could work openly without fear of prosecution.

Dissociation, the term that underlies the dissociative disorders including DID, lacks a precise, practical and generally agreed-upon definition. A large number of diverse experiences have been termed dissociative, ranging from normal failures in attention to breakdowns in the memory processes characterised by dissociative disorders. Therefore it's not known if there is a common root underlying dissociative experiences, or if the range of mild-to-severe symptoms is a result of different causes or origins, and biological structures. Other terms used include personality, personality state, identity, ego state and amnesia. They also have no agreed-upon definitions.

Basically, the psychiatrists and mental health clinicians haven't even come to an agreement as to what causes DID, let alone how to treat it. There will always be examples where people have other issues, which can confuse diagnosis. If the clinicians take into account the possible interference from the spirit world, their job would be a lot easier, and more people would get the help they need to deal with their specific condition. There is still much discussion and disagreement as to the cause and treatment of DID and until they consider the mind and brain as two separate things - one of the body and one of spirit - the final answer will continue to elude them.

It's stated in the Diagnostics and Statistical Manual of Mental Disorders (DSM) that DID includes "the presence of two or more distinct identities or personality states" that alternate control of the individual's behaviour. Individuals with DID may experience distress from both the symptoms of DID (intrusive thoughts or emotions) as well as the consequences of the accompanying symptoms (dissociation, rendering them unable to remember specific information). The identities appear to be unaware of each other and compartmentalise knowledge and memories, resulting in chaotic personal lives. Individuals with DID may be reluctant to discuss symptoms due to associations with abuse, shame and fear. The primary identity, which often has the patient's given name, tends to be "passive, dependent, guilty and depressed", while other personalities (or 'alters') are more active, aggressive or hostile and often contain more complete memories. Most identities are of ordinary people, but some pretend to be well- known individuals that have passed over. The most common form of complaint of DID is depression, with headaches being a common neurological symptom. A majority of those diagnosed with DID meet the criteria for DSM, with personality disorders such as borderline personality disorder. Further data supports a high level of psychotic symptoms in DID, and that both schizophrenia and DID have histories of trauma. People diagnosed with DID also demonstrate the highest hypnotisability of any clinical population. It is suggested that the large number of symptoms presented by people with DID is actually an indication of the severity of the other disorders diagnosed in the patient.

If you are being attacked and can't fight back, you would be depressed and fearful, as well as feeling guilty that you can't control things. The best form of defence is to attack, which is why the alters are usually aggressive or hostile. This is an invasion of the mind, nothing less, by intrusive thoughts or emotions: nobody asks where they're coming from. They are no different than the communication a medium gets, except the medium is able to control it. I have found that most people who suddenly become aware of spirit have had some kind of life-changing event prior to their spiritual experience, such as an accident, death of a loved one, losing a job, losing their home or partner, childhood abuse - the list goes on. Even puberty can cause emotional highs and lows, which is when you can become more sensitive to what's around you, seen and unseen.

People with DID are diagnosed with five to seven co-morbid

disorders on average, much higher than other mental illnesses. Due to overlapping symptoms, differential diagnosis includes schizophrenia, normal and rapid-cycling bi-polar disorder, epilepsy, borderline personality disorder and Asperger syndrome.

Before the nineteenth century, people exhibiting symptoms similar to DID were believed to be possessed. The first case history of DID, then known as Multiple personality disorder was written in great detail by Eberhardt Gmelin, in *A History of Dissociative Identity Disorder*. In the nineteenth century 'dedoublement' or double consciousness, the historical precursor to DID, was frequently described as a state of sleepwalking. Scholars hypothesised that the patients were switching between normal consciousness and a 'sonambulistic state'.

An intense interest in spiritualism, parapsychology and hypnosis continued throughout the nineteenth and twentieth centuries, running in parallel with John Locke's views that there was an association of ideas requiring the coexistence of feelings with awareness of feelings. Hypnosis, which was pioneered in the late nineteenth century by Franz Mesmer and Armand-Marie-Jacques de Chastenet, Marquis of Puysegur, challenged Locke's association of ideas. Hypnotists reported what they thought were second personalities emerging during hypnosis and wondered how the two minds could coexist.

There have been many discussions at international medical conferences, with no clear consensus other than it is a mental illness. There is still disagreement as to the cause and treatment of DID but it is generally agreed there are other mental illnesses running alongside the main condition.

It would appear they had the right idea in the 19th nineteenth century, but science overtook intuition. When under hypnosis it is very easy for a passing spirit to come through the patient's subconscious mind and relate their own story. This is one of the problems with regression - whose mind is providing the information, the patient's or the spirit's.

Spiritual Interference

People with dissociate identity disorder (DID), formerly known as multiple personality disorder (MPD), appear to have several different personalities that take control of the body and emerge separately. Some claim to be past life personalities, while others claim to be separate spirits and not part of the person.

While on our life's journey, we can pick up discarnate spirits who attach themselves to our aura or just stay close to us. If they have had an uncomfortable passing, through head injury or some other medical condition that causes pain, then just by staying close to us they can transmit the pain to us. Often when a person is sensitive they will pick up the pain as if it were their own. Even some symptoms of a disease can be transmitted to the person on the earth plane. So whether the spirit is attached or just close by really makes no difference: the result can be the same. There are some in spirit who purposely bring us pain or play on our emotions to gain control of us. We're not always aware that any of the above is not of our making; we just accept it, assuming it's our own condition.

Mediums used a mesmeriser to put themselves in a trancelike state, which is not unlike classic hypnosis. This is usually understood to be a sleep-like state that is induced by the hypnotist. In this hypnotic state, forgotten or suppressed memories can be experienced. Boredom or daydreaming can also bring on a hypnotic state, which is self-induced, but we're able to snap out of it by some outside stimulus. How often has time slipped by without us noticing, i.e. walking or driving and suddenly becoming aware of where we are and not remembering passing a certain point: it's not uncommon.

Hypnotherapists, are psychotherapists who use hypnosis to induce this mental state and ease chronic pain, or uncover upsetting memories that affect a person's life.

If a person talks about a past-life death, the past-life personality will remain intact simply because they are a discarnate spirit, who is talking about their own life and passing. All too often, it is thought the past-life entity is in fact relating the past life of the person who is undergoing therapy, when in fact they are two separate individuals. The fact is that the spirit who is relating their life and the traumas they suffered, doesn't realise in most cases that the host is suffering their pains. This does not stop the host from experiencing all the symptoms and discomforts the spirit has, or is suffering. By helping the entity to understand what has happened to them, and that the pain is of the body and not the spirit, the spirit will no longer feel the pain, and the discomfort will disappear from the person as the spirit moves into the light.

Most of the spirit attachments are benign and have no idea of the discomfort they may be causing the host. Once they have been given that understanding, they will often be very apologetic and move out of the host's aura into the light. There are those who have attached themselves so they can dictate, or even take over for short periods, the host's life. This is possession and it's been going on for centuries. It's recognised by many religions as evil spirits taking over someone's life, hence the exorcisms they perform. Unfortunately those who take possession are all deemed as evil in the eyes of the church, when in fact only a few are taking possession to gain control over the host. Most either don't realise the effect they're having, or it's a cry for help.

Mediumship is a form of voluntary possession, where the medium allows the spirit either to enter his body during trance, or influence his mind when giving messages. This is why mediums are more able to detect spirits around others, and help with possessions and hauntings.

William James, an eminent psychologist, seemed to accept the possibility of discarnate interference in a statement he made:

"The refusal of modern 'enlightenment' to treat possession as a hypothesis to be spoken of as even possible, in spite of massive human tradition based on concrete experiences in favour, has always seemed to me a curious example of power of fashion in things scientific. That the demon theory will have its innings again is to my mind absolutely certain. One has to be 'scientific' indeed be blind and ignorant enough to suspect no such possibility."

As has been said before, the scientific method will never be sufficient to explore thoroughly the depth of human consciousness. Research must include the spiritual dimensions.

Some specialist mediums deal with haunted houses and possession, but there are many mediums who don't believe in bad spirits or don't accept spirit can get lost even for a short time. Mediums have also been dealing with spirit attachments for years.

It can take quite a few sessions when dealing with malicious attachments, and sometimes even when they are persuaded to go, the host will feel empty and invite another to take their place. This is why it's important to make sure the host has an understanding of why they feel empty and that it will just be a brief time before they will feel themselves again. There are also problems which arise when a house is haunted by malevolent spirits who refuse to leave. Because the family living in the house have accepted that it's normal for them to have spirits around them, even if they're nasty, it takes education and strength of mind to overcome that acceptance. There are mediums who don't use trance or hypnosis to rescue souls, and they're usually able to converse directly with the spirit haunting a house. Unfortunately they don't always recognise or help people when they have attachments, because they aren't aware of them.

The Spiritual Point of View

It's a shame that the medical profession don't - or will not - accept there is another world that, although unseen to most, is still a reality. There are those who have passed over, who still want to communicate with this world, for one reason or another. Despite all the research that has been done, the profession steadfastly refuses to believe people can be influenced from beyond the grave. I wonder with all the psychic shows on television whether they think it's a trick. Do they just bury their heads in the sand, and blithely go along with the only rules they have for diagnosis? It's like putting people in boxes so they can categorise them and move on. Why they never consider the implications of mediumship as a possible avenue of research is beyond me. Maybe they feel it's not a science and as they can't touch or measure it, they discount it completely. It's surprising really, as a number of governments - including Russia and America - experimented with mediums during World War II, with a view to carry out remote-spying on each other.

Most psychiatrists and doctors seldom consider the soul or spirit as the cause of the problem, even if they accept its existence. It's a tragedy that many medical practitioners don't believe in the existence of the soul, and fail to recognise it as a possible health source. It's reflected in the tens of thousands of mentally ill patients, who needlessly live their lives in and out of mental institutions. The soul within is the origin of all our hopes and fears, and - like the body - it can be, and is, influenced by the world of spirit. This complex receptacle of the consciousness needs proper understanding, and will not be corrected by conventional medical techniques, as it is not of the organic brain but of the spirit. No-one should be left to suffer the sometimes devastating illnesses known to doctors as schizophrenia, DID and bi-polar disorder, where people are led from one emotion to another by the lack of understanding of the medical profession, and by friends and family.

With schizophrenia or spiritual interference, the interference and emotional changes can be quite severe, causing the individual to lose hope of trying to lead a 'normal' life. The daily routines become disrupted and often there are occasions when time seems to pass away without notice. Some get the feeling of being watched and indeed they are. But they can't work out by whom, so they become paranoid about their privacy. Gradually they withdraw from other people and the very fact that they isolate themselves only enhances their vulnerability to spirit interference. No age-group is immune (though older people take things in their stride more easily). Even children have imaginary friends but because they are innocent, they are easily persuaded that their 'friends' aren't real. People have been taken into deep depression by the havoc their emotions can play on them, and very serious consequences can arise, such as frequent thoughts of suicide and even acts of suicide and murder. How many times have we heard in the news that someone has been killed, because the perpetrator heard voices telling them to kill?

Researchers are obviously aware of the fact that spiritual depression is one of the most prevalent of psychic illnesses, but they continually fail to find medical reasons why it is happening, in spite of the most advanced analysis equipment and techniques. This clearly shows that the seat of the problem is beyond the physical. Advanced psychics and mystics are well aware of the fact because they, at one stage of their development, experience similar incapacitating disturbances, which originate in the mind, as opposed to the brain - a region not considered by psychiatrists, but well known to psychics as part of their pathway to enlightenment.

The brain is the physical organ that is responsible for the collection of data and day-to-day thoughts and experiences. It also controls basic functions like breathing and balance and registers pain in the body, regardless of how it occurs. The mind is where the emotions and feelings are and because the mind and brain work as one, it's difficult to divide the two processes. The mind is also the receptacle which stores information and is part of the soul or spirit, which also interacts with the spirit world on a subconscious level. It is only by developing the conscious mind that we are able to recognise some of what the subconscious mind is attuning to. The mind is also where we store life's experiences, which we take with us when we pass over. The mind can and sometimes does get conflicting information, when somebody is in this world but getting information from the spirit world. With no understanding of where the information is coming from, it can be very confusing, especially when others are not aware of the world of spirit.

For somebody suspected or diagnosed as schizophrenic, the frustrations and pains they undergo because of their sensitivity to the spirit world cause them to believe they are going mad. There seems to be no reason why they're suffering. The effects of these spiritual attacks are made even more terrifying by elements of ignorance and fear: there seems to be no obvious reason for them, or why they should be suffering these sometimes intense emotional changes, which cause despair and utter hopelessness. At times, they have a sneaking suspicion that they're heading for an irreversible mental breakdown or insanity. It makes it considerably more difficult for the medical profession, when trying to arrive at some diagnosis concerning a patient's ailment, when the true condition is often hidden or disguised by a number of physical symptoms such as headaches, stomach pains, tiredness, tension, and many other physical pains which can appear all over the body. Therefore the problem remains persistently active, but unrecognised by both the doctor and the patient. Once the exact nature of the illness, or more importantly the source, is understood, it will then become obvious to the researchers that some relief may be given by the use of drugs or psychoanalysis. But a permanent cure will never be found in the laboratory or chemists. Relief will be found only within the field so long ignored by psychiatrists - the mind.

The distinguishing factor concerning spiritual interference, is that the problem first presents itself when somebody is experiencing exceptional mood changes. These can lead to feelings of sadness and hopelessness, characterised by recurrent pains and discomfort. The frequency of these attacks, and their lack of understanding as to why they are feeling these pains, can leave them baffled and full of fear. The first important approach is to help the sufferer understand how and why they are being attacked. This will gradually lead to a slow decrease in the frequency of the attacks. They will begin to feel better about themselves and realise that they are not at fault, by gradually being helped to understand the nature of their problem. With patience and perseverance they can gradually build up their stability, but this is only the beginning of a long and difficult struggle. The more knowledge that can be given, the more stable they will become, until finally they are able to control the attacks of the body through the mind.

The greatest problem with which they have to cope is the emotional pain and lack of understanding these attacks can bring. These can be so intense, in some cases, that they present a real psychiatric emergency. It is among these people that suicide presents the highest risk. With spiritual interference, they are convinced that life has radically changed and it will never be the same, as they will always hear or see things others don't. This is true, but by understanding what is happening they are able, over time, to control what is happening. Their behaviour is generally withdrawn with a feeling of fatigue and often is interrupted by bouts of abuse and aggression. Other outward signs include appearing to talk to themselves, sudden mood changes and disturbed sleep, a total disinterest in socialising, and low self-esteem.

Another problem that they have to face is the fear that, periodically, something takes control of their conscious and subconscious thoughts, and they don't know what's going to happen next. They lose time and awareness of their surroundings, and are sometimes completely unaware of what they're doing or saying. This is not only demoralising but adds greatly to the risk of suicide. It arises simply through their inability to understand what's happening to them. Fear, being the most imaginative of our emotions, thrusts into the mind thoughts of impending insanity, evil possession and brain damage. This fear is very real to them, because they are unable to separate their own thoughts and actions from those given to them from the spirit realms.

The material situation - such as family affairs, occupation, finance and physical health - are usually reasonably sound in the beginning, and there seems to be no reason why they are being attacked. Therefore it's a case of ignorance adding substantially to the problem. Once they understand the exact nature of the attacks, only then will it be realised that drugs, shock treatment and psychoanalysis cannot possibly help the problem. So far, medical science, after years of research, has not produced any results which show promise of a cure. It's extremely unlikely that one will be found by pursuing much the same theoretical medical beliefs.

Having to suffer these disturbing mental attacks day after day without understanding why they're happening; having nothing else to turn to but the routine medication, which produces piteously few signs of progress, can leave them in a zombie-like existence (all the while they are taking the prescribed medication) for the rest of their lives. In addition, the medication or treatment, which is not a cure, can damage the brain.

Lack of knowledge is the key. Not knowing how or why creates a frightening private hell. Therefore, the first step towards establishing some degree of stability is to replace ignorance with knowledge. To succeed in helping someone is to give them an understanding of the problem and the reasons why it's happening to them, is the beginning of getting their mind back under control. We can then work towards a slow but certain build-up towards a mental stability. Greater understanding will then lead to the ability to control one's thoughts and actions.

I have always believed that we live in a world where there is interaction with those who have passed before us. Unfortunately those who have passed into the spirit world are not always benign. They will often have issues which they need to address and sometimes they will interfere with those left on the earth plane. It's this interaction that can cause mental and psychological problems for those sensitive individuals they interact with. By understanding the nature of the problem, most people can - and do - come to terms with it and are able to control their minds. It's not an easy journey at first, but with guidance and practice, it can be achieved. Understanding what the spirit world can do and how far some will go is the beginning of getting the mind under control. Unfortunately there are few who work in this field who understand the ramifications of this spirit interaction. The medical profession tries to treat the symptoms, but will never succeed until it recognises the cause of the problem.

Understanding

It's important to understand that it's not an easy task which the medium is about to embark on. When a medium allocates time to someone, teaching them to understand, and encouraging them to stick rigidly to the advice and mental exercises suggested, there can be no turning back or giving up by either party if the end result is to be achieved. It can take months and they must show courage and determination to face and resist the attacks and demands of those in the spirit realms.

Take the case of Terri - his name has been changed to protect his privacy

The initial approach of the medium is most important. A strong rapport with the person is vital to preparing the basis for the education that is to follow. This is achieved by first allowing Terri to talk without interruption and explain what's going on, so that I can understand how she is aware of the attacks. It's important to understand how Terri perceives her situation and not to discredit any of her statements at this early stage, so that I can understand the scope of Terri's knowledge of her situation. By listening carefully to what is being said, I give Terri a sense of confidence, and so draw out some of the things that otherwise may not be mentioned, as Terri may consider them trivial. Everything relating to the problem is important and it's my job as the medium to understand from Terri's point of view. It's important to work within her understanding and not belittle her beliefs and experiences.

I would not try to rush things, as Terri must be given the chance to understand why it's happening to her. She needs to hear the reasons why she is getting attacked and how it's happening. The object of the exercise is to replace the terrors of ignorance with understanding of the reason she has been singled out. Not knowing why she is being subjected daily to these demoralising attacks breeds fear and despair. Terri needs to recognise and understand the pattern of the attacks and the reasons behind them. This will slowly but substantially build up a mental stability, from which I can proceed towards getting things under control.

Terri must practise and repeat the mental exercises until they become second nature. She must be taught to fight back and not just think of herself as a helpless, powerless victim against these attacks: the attacks will become more controllable over time. At every opportunity, I would impress upon Terri the crucial point that the most valuable moment for her to fight back is at the beginning of, or during an, attack.

It will not be an easy task that I am asking Terri to undertake. It will call for tremendous patience and determination, concentration and courage. Even if these qualities are brought to bear upon the problem for only brief moments, some advance towards relief and ultimate control of the mind will be achieved. Once started, I would impress upon Terri that there is no going back, as to give up would mean the attacks would become a way of life with no escape. The only way to achieve mental and emotional harmony is to see it through to the end. Terri would be made aware of this from the beginning and continuously encouraged to fight on. It's a battle of wills and Terri must be aware of what she is getting into before she takes up the fight. Terri will have to play the biggest part in her recovery and there will be times when she is unable to take control. But ultimately if she fights on, the attacks will become less of a problem, until they eventually become no more than a minor irritation.

If Terri is sincere and determined to free herself from these distressing attacks she must be prepared to defend herself, initially many times a day, using the mental exercises which she has been taught. However tedious these may be, Terri must be suitably careful and recognise them as the only effective methods available to find peace of mind.

Getting the Mind Under control

We are all given the choice of responsibility: whether we use it or not is up to the individual. By allowing others to influence us, we allow them to take away our free will to choose. We are all individually responsible for what we allow to happen in our lives and we can make a choice or not. If we refuse to be accountable for what happens to us, then we have only ourselves to blame. The problem is that until we make a stand, and refuse to accept interference from whatever source, we don't realise the power we have given others to control us. We can carry negative feelings all through our lives and if we don't deal with them, this can lead to low esteem and self-worth. Spiritually we are all born equal, but as we grow so we allow others to set our pathway through life. We must take responsibility for our 'self' or we will be puppets for whoever exerts their will on us. If we look back on our life, we will see how we have been influenced by others, sometimes for our benefit, but many times to our detriment. There are occasions when it's obvious who is trying to influence us and other times when it's not. We just get a feeling that we should or shouldn't do something: is that our mind or is that outside interference? Ignorance of the spirit realms is no excuse; we must follow our instincts from the beginning.

Our beliefs keep us chained to an idea which, although it may not be true, will stop us from examining other possibilities and ways to free ourselves. If we are rigid in our thinking, then we will be kept captive by our own thoughts and beliefs. This is particularly so of science and religion; we must examine all possibilities so we can free our minds and take back the responsibility to decide for ourselves. It's no good saying it is so because it always has been - if mankind had done that we would still be in the Stone Age. It's the same with spirituality - for thousands of years mankind has known instinctively that life goes on in another way after death, yet it's only now that we are looking more closely at the effects those who have gone before us can have on our lives.

Focussing the mind is where I taught Terri exercises that will help her to control her thoughts and block any unwanted images and thoughts from her mind. I will achieve this by showing Terri certain exercises which she will need to practise daily. There will always be one or two people who will not be able to accept this mental discipline. They will resign themselves to the idea that there is no escape for them from the mental interference. To those people, I can only say that I have found no other way except the way I'm putting before you.

The principle objective of self-discipline is to bring the thoughts, images and feelings under Terri's own control, giving her the ability to override the thoughts and images that are put into her mind by those in the spirit realms. By understanding her own capabilities, she will gain strength and encouragement which will help her to bring her life back under control.

There are many techniques to bring the mind under control and all of these have much the same objective in common. I will set out two of these, as too many will lead to confusion and might be self-defeating. Whichever technique is used, it must be adaptable to Terri's circumstances, although the basics will remain the same. It is essential that it be carefully followed and practised regularly without change, until It fine-tune the technique for Terri's individual circumstances that are being dealt with. While bearing in mind that Terri is embarking on a course of mental discipline, it should be noted that there are those in the spirit world who will try to interfere with the process. By giving Terri negative thoughts and believable reasons as to why she shouldn't start the meditation, and why it should be put off, and interrupting at every opportunity, they're fighting to keep control and will try anything to stop Terri from removing them. The golden rule to observe at all times is, when any reason enters the mind suggesting ending or suspending the practice, whether it be tiredness or some other outer attraction, to recognise it to be a subtle diversion and persevere with the routine.

The greatest difficulty which confronts Terri will be her inability to focus the mind and concentrate on the exercise being practised. Most minds are invaded by stray thoughts, emotions, fears and random ideas which wander in and out. If the mind is completely under the control of the will, instead of it behaving like a piece of paper in a strong wind, Terri will be firmly on the way to stability and control. You might like to test the restless and impulsive nature of your everyday mind with this simple experiment. Fix in your mind's eye an ordinary object like a matchstick or a flower, attempt to hold the image steady in the focus of the mind's eye for 10 or 20 seconds. You will inevitably fail because the image will have been, almost unnoticeably, replaced by another different thought. Try again with another experiment. Try to keep the mind completely free of any thought for 10 seconds. The same failure will result.

Despite your most valiant efforts, the unfortunate fact is that the conscious efforts themselves have become thoughts, which are throwing the mind off-course, in their own silent way. When people eventually realises this they then try other disciplinary techniques until their mind is so cluttered up with such a mass of concepts, they finally give up to the mounting frustration. The damage is done when effort is applied with strain.

The ideal approach to a thought-free mind is a slow one, through concentration: this is the first stage and it must be practised without thinking. First sit comfortably in a chair, preferably a dining chair because if you make yourself too comfortable you may fall asleep. Begin the concentration on a simple image such as a matchstick or a flower. Hold this picture in the mind's eye, relax the mind and calmly note the image's shape and colour. When you find yourself thinking about something else, as is to be expected, gently remove the thought and replace the image. A word of warning: beware of the spirits' favourite deterrent, impatience. Be prepared to sit for many weeks and expect very little to happen at first. With practice you will start to hold the image longer. You mustn't look for success - it will come in its own time with practice. You must have confidence; as an experienced traveller on this particular discipline, I know you will achieve your goal over time if you practise daily.

For those who find the practice or direct-image-concentration difficult, because of their inability to deal with the many distractions, there is an alternative - the creative visuals technique. With this method the person is encouraged to think using the faculty of imagination and the memory-trains of four of the five senses; smell, touch, sight and hearing. This is how to begin: again sit in a chair which is not too comfortable - a dining chair is ideal. You should imagine you're walking along a towpath beside a canal. With this technique, instead of trying to make your mind blank you actually concentrate and fill the mind with pictures. Visualise the canal and the towpath, see the surrounding trees or hedges. Notice the flowers, and whether there are any ducks or swans. Now look up and study the clouds and birds flying above.. Allow your imagination to paint a picture that is comfortable Take notice of the leaves and their colours - this will give you a sense of the time of year.

So far you have only used sight. You can now move on to combine hearing with your observations: Listen can you hear the birds and is there a breeze rustling the leaves? As you listen, you may hear in the distance a dog bark, or the sound of farm animals. While listening to the different sounds, continue to visualise - can you feel the stones beneath your feet or feel a breeze on your face? Smell the grass in the nearby field. You have now succeeded in combining sight, touch, hearing and smell in this exercise.

This meditative technique is very different from mere mind wandering, because you are intentionally directing the mind in a disciplined way, while using the faculty of imagination, which is also a form of mind discipline.

These exercises in concentration are two of the most fundamental in all mental disciplines. They will ultimately enable you to detach yourself, at will, from the attacks on your consciousness by those in spirit. By putting your own thoughts in your mind, you will be able to block out these extraneous thoughts and feelings from the spirit realms.

By learning to focus the mind, the person is able to block unwanted thoughts and pictures by focussing on their own images. It's an incredibly difficult and challenging road you will have to travel, and at times you may fail, but the important thing is to get up and try again, because with perseverance you will succeed.

Gaining control of the mind is the first step in the long journey to freeing yourself from interference. Once this is achieved, it is then time to work on the feelings that are received, be they emotional or physical. It's easy for spirit to affect the person's emotions by putting doubts into the mind which the person will - with a bit of prodding - escalate out of all proportion. The thought may have no basis, but it can be built on by continuous nagging from spirit, so that it appears to be a reality. It's important to learn to recognise these thoughts which are not your own and squash them as soon as they're recognised. By using the aforementioned techniques, the mind can be controlled and unwanted feelings and thoughts can be blocked. When pain is received it's important to consider whether it's the result of something the person has done or it's reasonable to expect, such as a hangover if they have drunk too much, or pain if they have banged their arm. Pain can be given by those in spirit to distract or control. When spirit gives pain it's a memory of what the person or the spirit has suffered in the past that is being brought back to the conscious mind. Sometimes if the spirit is feeling pain, the person may pick up their feelings but if you recognise it to be alien to yourself, it will go away. You can never be given a disease or ailment you have never had - but they can give you the symptoms and also make a current problem seem worse. If the person has no reason to have the pain, then they should repeatedly tell themselves it's not theirs, and it will go away. If it persists, then for ease of mind take the appropriate medication and continue to practise the techniques that have been suggested. The more proficient the person becomes, the more they will understand how to deal with negative spiritual interference.

Possession

There has been great interest by medical science in the cause and treatment of psychological illnesses. The statistics show that mental disorders are increasing alarmingly in most countries around the world. Yet medical scientists are no nearer to understanding the causes than they were 100 years ago.

Though the world's leading researchers in psychiatry and neurology differ widely in their theories regarding the origin of certain mental abnormalities, they still believe the primary cause is a physically malfunctioning nervous system or brain. Scientists may not be aware of the exact causes of mental disorders, but it is a documented fact that insanity and other psychological disorders are totally devoid of any physical deterioration of the brain. Mental health specialists have said that brain damage or tumours may create physical impediments, but they have never been known to directly affect the mind. In other words there may be damage to the physical brain causing physical problems, but the individuals still retain a perfectly normal mind. Therefore the mind abnormality must be due to some influence from outside the brain. So the mind must be affected by some invisible source outside the body.

Since animal, vegetable and mineral - as science has proved - is nothing more than energy in constant motion, in other words visible nature, it is therefore difficult for most to accept that their physical existence and that of their visible, tangible, world is completely dependent on invisible elements and forces. When we realise that every aspect of visible nature is only an intricate combination of invisible energies and frequencies, the existence of other energies beyond the visible frequencies becomes acceptable, for example a world where spirit forms exist without physical form, invisible to all who are not sensitive to the spirit frequencies.

If we look at the historical findings of early races, we will see that as far back as can be traced, dedication to the spirits of the departed was the earliest form of worship. Definite ideas of the human soul or spirit were recorded by primitive tribes all over the world, and there was a belief in the continuance of their ancestors beyond bodily death. Many classical teachings of philosophers such as Plato and Socrates refer to spirit existence as an established fact. The majority of the world's religious works, including the Old and New Testaments, are full of references to the continuation of the consciousness. Over the past two hundred years there have been many investigations into the afterlife. Evidential proof has been compiled during these investigations by prominent scientists and philosophers such as Sir William Crooks, Sir Oliver Lodge, William Wallace and countless other scientists and philosophers throughout the world. Because the spirit realms have a different energy frequency, it interpenetrates with our own world without interference. It would not be thought of as an intangible world to those who exist there: it's as real and solid to them as is our own to us. There is a continuance of life here, but with certain natural and important differences. On earth our main responsibility is to sustain the body in an environment agreeable to our body's requirements. Knowledge and understanding comes to us through continuous experiences of the many physical laws we encounter in our daily lives. For most, the race of life was the long struggle against hardships, suffering and tragedy simply to preserve life or maintain ourselves in a comfortable relationship with our surroundings.

On the spirit plane, we no longer need to eat or sleep and this takes away the continuous struggle for survival. The soul still has the desire to progress, but the mind unfolds, for many, along different lines. There is no longer the need to conform to others' expectations. Once the mind is awakened from the long conditioned earthly state and looks around at the new world, it realises that it's all too familiar: earthly consciousness is deeply rooted in a spiritual level. The meaning and purpose of existence becomes all too clear and so real that the two basic fears that dominated our earthly existence, the fear of losing our possessions and the fear of not getting that which we desired, no longer exist.

The spirit world, with its more decisive and active thought force, gives us glimpses of a new quality of consciousness which ultimately provides an instrument that is increasingly more efficient and responsive, for the further advancement of the consciousness. Therefore the mind is inspired to unfold along lines of higher ideals, encouraged by the ever-widening conception of life's purpose.

The earth had acted as a veil, preventing us from understanding the true nature and purpose of life, although for some mystics, prophets and mediums, that veil has become partly transparent and they are able to see something of the spirit realms. The act of passing from the physical to the spiritual world does not change the state of the mind of the individual; the soul remains as before. After 'death' the individual still carries their earthly habits, faults, beliefs and disbeliefs. By understanding this, we realise that those who led destructive lives are often determined to carry on with their destructive ideas. Apart from those malicious souls, there are earthbound spirits who, for one reason or another, have not learnt to progress from one plane to another, with the result that some become parasitic upon those left behind, simply because they don't know any better. There are also those who know exactly where they are, and take advantage of their new-found anonymity to annoy those who are sensitive enough to be affected by them.

There are also innocent souls who are in torment or lost for many reasons - from a belief or lack of belief in the hereafter, to not knowing they have died. Sometimes their only way of attracting attention to their plight is to make themselves known to individuals on the earth plane. They don't mean to cause distress, but by making their presence felt they can unwittingly cause suffering and worry.

There are plenty of documented cases of possession by what are termed devils of human origin through all ages and cultures. In fact the Bible has numerous accounts of possession by unclean or evil spirits, and the people of the times thought if they could cast out these spirits by performing exorcisms, they would attain the state of disciples. In fact most of the works of Jesus were described as casting out demons or unclean spirits. The films we see about hauntings are just that, dramatised for effect. Spirits don't make heads spin round or bodies float off the bed, but they can and do take possession of the body through the mind and control speech and actions.

There have been prolonged worldwide scientific studies to try to understand the unseen force of spirit phenomena. Scientists finally had to admit that it was no longer possible to push psychic phenomena to one side as a myth. The church has always accepted the existence and the reality of spiritualistic and evil external intelligences. However, even today they have been unable to define the nature and source of the intelligence. Whenever there is a case of the creation of stress and mental confusion and suffering, the answer has always been classify it as diabolical possession and use the standard set of rules set out by the church for exorcism. All invasions of the mind were accepted as the actions of evil spirits of a vengeful nature. It was never considered a possibility that it might be a seriously disorientated human being in spirit form, desperately trying to attract attention to their dilemma.

It's becoming commonplace for an experienced medium or psychic to help rehabilitate distressed spirits, and it demands a more thorough understanding of the problem and much more patience when dealing with this kind of problem. The procedure to follow is to talk to the spirit and help them to understand their exact circumstances, and help them to come to terms with their situation, and help them to move on to the world of spirit. Although possession is caused by discarnate spirits, it is important to differentiate it from obsession, which is often used by doctors, psychiatrists and some psychical researchers to describe abnormal behaviour. Obsession is purely psychological, not a psychic problem, which has as its underlying cause a recurring, usually distressing, thought which has been deeply implanted in the brain by a dramatic or traumatic experience or series of events. The mental balance of an obsessional patient may be simply and fully restored by a course of psychoanalysis conducted by a competent psychiatrist, whereas to remove a possessing spirit a fully experienced and often courageous medium is required.

It's no surprise that the scientific approach to curing possession doesn't work. The doctors and psychiatrists haven't understood the difference, nor even considered that there may be something other than the brain which is causing the patient so much distress.

Although the latest World Health Organisation figures show an alarming increase in cases of insanity and are still rising, there are still a great number of neurologists and psychiatrists who believe that all causes of insanity lie somewhere in a deranged mental system. Doctors attempt to explain the fact that there is no difference in the brain of an insane person and that of a normal person. They believe an unknown organism or subtle chemical imbalance, which is as yet undetected, is causing the problem. They continue to believe in something regardless of the evidence that has been produced by eminent researchers into paranormal and psychic phenomena. They do so even to the extent that one prominent brain consultant said: "Something causes insanity but we have no idea what it is." It's time the neurologists and psychiatrists started listening to the mediums and psychic researchers.

For a lot of highly active neuroses, doctors admit that no definition exists and no anatomy is available to give guidance, simply because for most forms of functional derangement no pathological anatomy can be found. Therefore, after careful examination of all applied normal and abnormal psychological and pathological tests, and their subsequent elimination, when all results have been classified there still remains a very wide area of mental abnormality which cannot be explained by standard methods of research.

That long-established and highly experienced authorities largely disagree among themselves and cannot accurately and conclusively define the cause of these mental aberrations surely is strong reason, in view of the seriousness of the problem, for them to look into the possibility of man being a duality - matter and spirit - and the further possibility that certain people can be subjected to spirit interference.

This, therefore, must establish some grounds for the belief that impingement upon earthly living persons by outside influences is not only highly possible but has been demonstrated hundreds of times by psychics or mediums who have successfully released earthbound spirits who are influencing certain people.

It's not only lost or tormented souls who communicate. On a daily basis, mediums also provide evidence of survival, quite apart from releasing lost souls, when they communicate with a loved one who has died.

Since research into paranormal activities has become so widespread, physical science has been totally inadequate in the search to find complete answers regarding the true nature of ourselves. The hypothesis for paranormal activities, which includes the problem of possession, has advanced to a point where it should soon rank as a scientific subject. The mountain of evidence of paranormal activity grows daily, contributed to by some of the most eminent in science and medicine. This makes it increasingly certain in the near future that those concerned with mental health will wake up, not only to the fact that possession of the living by the invisible 'dead' is largely the cause of insanity, but that an amazing new field of research is open to them which will completely change the treatment of the mentally unbalanced.

Because the cause of many mental illnesses still eludes the world's leading neurologists and psychiatrists, despite their prolonged research programmes, this only adds dramatically to the call for help on behalf of thousands of people miserably locked up in mental institutions, that they should now turn their attentions and skills to spiritual science. They would then accept that insanity and other mental disturbances could be psychic neuroses. In which case, trained mediums should be introduced into the wards, laboratories and even our prisons.

We have established, on more than just reasonable grounds, the belief that the human personality survives physical death; that it's possible, given certain conditions, for the deceased person to communicate through a medium, or - if spiritually uneducated - invade the physical body of someone living on earth. When all possible alternatives have been examined, double-checked and exhausted, there will still remain a surplus of evidence that can't possibly be explained except by the survival and possession hypothesis. This residue is so widespread, that it's remarkable that psychiatrists haven't at least considered this untapped field in their search for answers to those functional neuroses which defy definition and conventional treatment.

It has been obvious to many mediums that schizophrenia is caused by interference from the spirit world, and therefore has nothing to do with the organic brain but rather the mind, which is influenced by discarnate spirits. This surely indicates beyond doubt that the human personality survives physical death; that it is possible, given certain conditions, for the discarnate spirit to communicate via a medium, or to invade the ethereal body of someone living on earth. There are many hundreds of thousands of people who suffer from schizophrenia needlessly because of the medical professions' stubbornness to explore the obvious possibilities that have been staring them in the face for hundreds of years.

The following are some case studies taken from our files where we came across people either exhibiting schizophrenic symptoms, or who had been diagnosed as having paranoid schizophrenia. All cases were displaying similar problems, which were originating from the spiritual realms. Sometimes we were able to deal with the problem in one sitting but at other times it could take many visits. I have selected some cases that demonstrate why it isn't always a quick fix and that it can take months to free people of interference. I have also added a case where we were unable to help and the reasons why.

Case 2

It was in August 2000 that I met Rose at a church where I was running a closed circle. One of the sitters asked if it would be okay for her to join us.

As Rose had sat in circle before and a couple of sitters were unable to attend anymore, I said 'yes that would be fine'. During the closed circle I studied Rose to make sure she was the right person to sit in a closed circle. She seemed a bit unsettled and I thought at first it was because it was her first night among strangers. During the circle I realised there was more to it than that, but decided to let things ride for the moment and just monitor the situation. When we sat the following week, Rose seemed a little more at ease and did quite well for her second time with us. Although she seemed to be settling down I was aware there was something more going on - Rose had a tendency to lose her words or struggle to find the right words when she was giving clairvoyance, yet at other times had no difficulty in speaking. She also had a nervous habit of twitching her fingers or rubbing her hands while working. It was obvious she wasn't sleeping properly because she had a sort of haunted look in her eyes.

On the third week, while in meditation, Rose became aware of an individual who was said he was her spirit guide. I was aware of this because during the meditation, which I talk through, I focus on each sitter to make sure they're alright and to see who they have with them. After the meditation I go round the circle and discuss who they had with them and how they felt. If we differ in the information we get, then we discuss it further. I explain what they got and why they got something different from me, so they understand how they missed the more subtle things that were happening.

When I got round to Rose, I asked her:

"What were you aware of?"

"I was aware of a monk who came forward."

I never tell the sitters who I am aware of, as they may not know that particular guide, and it may not be time yet. I always ask who they are aware of and then I tune in to whoever they get and check them out.

I focussed on to the monk and asked her a few questions

about how he looked and what he wore. What she told me agreed with what I was getting, apart from the colour of his clothes. I still felt something wasn't right, so I asked her:

"How were you aware of him, and how did he make his presence known?"

"I closed my eyes and he was there all of a sudden - as large as life."

"Has he always shown himself to you in that way?"

"No, sometimes he comes in slowly and sometimes he's there already."

"I see - and what was he wearing?"

"Sometimes he's dressed in an off-white habit and sometimes it's brown."

"Your guides will always show themselves wearing the same thing, and will only ever come in slowly, never just appear. When he comes in a brown habit, how do you feel?"

"Okay, but it's not the same as the other times when he's dressed in off-white."

"When he comes in dressed in the brown habit, does he always come in suddenly?"

"I'm not sure, I think so - I've never taken that much notice."

"How do you feel when he comes in like that?"

"Usually I feel a little agitated."

"When the monk in off-white comes in, do you feel calmer?"

"Yes and more at ease too."

"Now you see the difference between what's right and what's not. The monk in brown is an imposter, trying to mislead you and keep you from getting to know your real guides."

"Why would anyone want to stop me from getting to know my guides?"

"There are those in the spirit realms that are not qualified or experienced enough to take on the role of guide. A guide is a very experienced spirit who you ask to look after you while you're there. You choose them from amongst your friends while you're in spirit, for their abilities and expertise. They're there to help you to understand your journey through life, and to advise and protect you. They're bound by the rule of free will, so cannot interfere with your choices. The reason we sit in circles is so that those of us who are more experienced at tuning-in to guides can help others learn the right way to do things. You must remember that if you're going to work with spirit, then you'll want to work with the right people in spirit, to achieve the best results you can for those you go on to help in the future.

"There are those who will want to mislead you and interfere with your choices. They don't have the expertise or the knowledge to help you, or any intention of doing anything but furthering their own aims. If they can stop you getting to know your guides, then they may be able to get you to themselves. If that happens, then you will be at their beck and call whenever they choose. They will interfere with your sleep and your daily life by making demands, or encouraging you to give information to someone who hasn't asked you to contact spirit. This can be upsetting for people and you will be labelled as mentally ill or just plain mad. Once they get you, it's difficult to get rid of them, and if you need help there are very few people who know how to deal with it."

"So what you're saying is that even in circle they're there trying to interfere. Why do our guides let them? Why don't they stop them coming to our circle? After all, we always open in prayer and ask for protection," Rose said.

"Your guides are restricted by free will - if you choose to listen to those who are not guides, then they must abide by your decision, as one of their prime roles is non- interference. As for opening in prayer, what's a prayer? You'll probably say you're sending thoughts to a higher being, asking for protection, and so as you have asked, you will receive. Well it's not for me to tell you who to pray to, but would you consider that as your guides have dedicated themselves to assisting you while you're here, wouldn't it be a good idea to pray or talk to them? Maybe there is a higher being - I really couldn't say at this stage, but if there was, wouldn't your guides be working for him/her? As they're your first contact with the spirit realms, it would be best to get to know them - after all, these guides are who you'll be working with spiritually."

"Yes I see what you're saying, but I had never thought of it like that before. So the monk in the brown habit is trying to mislead me?"

"Yes, so when he comes forward you can either throw him out if you can, or alternatively open your eyes. As you get to know your real guide, the monk in the brown habit will stop coming because you will gradually build an affinity with your monk in off-white and naturally block out the other one."

"Why do our guides allow this sort of thing to happen? If, as you say, we're praying to our guides, don't they listen when we ask for protection and stop the imposters from coming in?"

"Again it's about free will - if they don't let the wrong ones come forward, how will you know what's right and what's wrong? It's only by experience that you learn to tell the difference. As you've just seen, although you were feeling agitated, you were not sure if the monk in brown was right or wrong. By comparing the feelings you get from the imposter and the monk in off-white, you can clearly see how different it feels."

"What about when mediums say 'like attracts like' - doesn't that mean that if you're a good person then you will only attract good spirits?"

"It's no different in spirit than it is here. How many nasty people have you met in your lifetime? Yet you consider yourself to be a good person, don't you?"

"Yes I see what you mean - nothing changes just because you go to spirit."

"Well yes it does. When you go to spirit then you'll adjust to the ways of the world you find yourself in, and when you get your spiritual memory back, you'll know just who you are. It's in the spirit realms around the earth where things don't really change for you, because you don't meet your loved ones or your guides, (because you don't see them) and you're not able to access your spiritual memory. Most people go straight to spirit, but there are some who get lost - they're the ones stuck in the spirit realms around the earth. Not all earthbound spirits are bad, but usually when we're developing as mediums, they're the ones who try to contact us or interfere. They still want to communicate with those of us on the earth, and live our lives for us in some cases. Part of a medium's development is to learn to tell who is a loved one by the feelings they're giving and the affinity we feel with the recipient when giving communication.

When we were nearly at the conclusion of the circle, Rose started to get upset. I had been hoping she would be able to control the feelings she had been getting. Throughout the circle, she had been bothered by the monk in brown. He was not going to give up easily. He tried a few times to influence her when she was trying to tune in to other things. She had a few tears. I asked her.

"What's wrong?"

Rose said: "I've been trying to block out the other monk all night, but he just keeps making me feel miserable. I know I'm not, but I just keep getting the feeling that I want to cry."

"If I can give you some healing, I'll get rid of him for you."

"Yes please," she said.

I went over to her and stood behind her and placed my hands on her shoulders. I could feel the monk with her and asked my guides to assist me in removing him. After a couple of minutes Rose started to feel better and when I'd finished she was visibly brighter, as though a great weight had been lifted from her shoulders. I asked her.

"How're you feeling now?"

"I feel much better - what did you do?"

"We call it an extraction. When someone is having trouble getting rid of unwanted spirits, I ask my guides to help me and they remove the spirit from you. They then talk to the spirit and try to make them see they're doing wrong. In some cases they are able to persuade them to go to the light. Others who refuse to leave, they have to remove and place them in a bubble of light so they can feel the energy from the spirit world. Usually, after a while, the spirit feels the calm and the warmth in the light and chooses to go to spirit."

"Will he come back?"

"No, he can't - we've put an energy around him and placed protection around you. Your positive protection will repel his negative energy, so he won't be able to get near you again. There are, however, other spirits who will try to imitate him."

"Why should that protection work if it doesn't when we ask for protection round the circle?"

"It does work when it's put round the circle. Because it's a learning situation, your guides allow you to pick up what's outside the protection. If you do that then they will let whatever you pick up come in, so you can learn from it. Your guides will never give you something bad or uncomfortable, so they let the negative spirits in to give you that kind of experience. They will never allow more than you can cope with to come in - sometimes you will feel you're getting more than you can handle, but you will always come through. You may think you don't want it anymore, but they are only helping you to learn the lessons you came here for. I know it doesn't help not knowing why you're here, but rest assured it will all make sense one day."

After the circle, I asked Rose:

"Have you had this problem before?"

"Yes but it's not only in circle - it's anytime. Suddenly I feel miserable or depressed and it takes me ages to sort myself out again."

"Are you having problems sleeping?" I asked.

"Yes, I haven't had a good night's sleep in ages."

I was aware there were still negative spirits around her and asked:

"Are you very tired when you go to bed, but as soon as you lie down, you feel wide awake?"

"Yes," she said.

"Do you get sudden mood-changes for no apparent reason?"

"Yes."

"Do you also get sudden pains like headaches and stomach aches?"

Rose looked surprised and said: "Yes - how did you know?"

"You're being attacked by negative earthbound spirits. They'll latch onto an individual just to make their life a misery. It's not just in circle or with spiritualists, it's anyone they can get to. How long has this been going on?"

"It's been going on for as long as I can remember. How do you know it's nasty spirits?"

"I can see and feel them around you. When you come to the church, do you have an argument with yourself about coming?"

"Yes I do, one minute I think I've made up my mind and then I'm not sure. Sometimes it's difficult to leave the house to come here."

"Do you find it difficult to leave the house on other occasions too?"

"Yes, it's like I'm frightened of open spaces. I know I'm not, but it feels that way sometimes."

"I think, if you would like, I will help you to get rid of these nasty spirits."

"How would you do that?"

"I will come to your house, with a few people who I work with, and remove them."

"So it's as simple as that?"

"It can be, but it all depends on how much of a hold they have on you. How long it will take to get you completely clear of them depends on how much influence they have over you. It will also depend on how you understand what has been going on, and how long it takes for you to understand how to protect yourself."

"How will I know how to protect myself?"

"I'll teach you and explain what's going on as we go along."

"That would be fine, when can you come round?"

"I'll arrange it with my friends and let you know. We'll come to a convenient time that suits us all - is that alright?"

"Yes, I'll give you my number. Thanks."

I asked Rose if it was alright to bring all the circle, as it would be the first time for some of them.

"Yes that would be fine," she said.

I spoke to some of the people who I work with in the rescue circle, and asked if they would like to go. They were keen to put their training into practice. This was their first time at someone's house. We sorted out a night when we were all available. I contacted Rose and made arrangements for the following Friday.

When Rose went to the doctor, she had been given tranquillisers which she didn't need, so she weaned herself off them before coming to the spiritualist church. If she had pursued that avenue and gone back to the doctor's, she would almost certainly have been referred to a psychiatrist for evaluation. He would most probably have diagnosed Rose as schizophrenic and I shudder to think what he would have given her as treatment.

Confronting the Spirits

On the way to Rose's house, I explained to my friends that they were not to open up, and should follow my instructions throughout and all would be well.

When we arrived, Rose was a bit apprehensive as she didn't know anyone except me, but after the introductions she settled down a bit.

I explained to everyone how we were going to go about it.

I said: "I'll check the house out and see where the spirits are. Then I'll ask one of you to go into trance and bring one of them through. I'll describe who I want you to get. When you bring them through, we'll talk to them and deal with them according to their situation. Rose - if at any time you feel uncomfortable in any way, let me know, okay?"

"Okay," Rose said.

All were agreed, so when everyone was settled I checked the house out and came back and sat down.

"There's a man about five foot seven with black hair and he's quite a fat man, he's not very nice, so be prepared for some horrible feelings. He'll try to put you off so you'll let him go. Do what you've been doing in the circle and everything will be alright."

I asked one of the light-trance mediums to tune in to him, and when she gave me more of his description, I knew she had the right person, so asked her to bring him through.

"Good evening," I said.

"Who are you and what do you want?" he asked.

"I've brought you through so that I can have a chat about what you're doing here."

"That's none of your business. I have nothing to say to you - go away."

"Well that's not very nice," I said. "We've come to find out why you're upsetting the lady and to sort out the problems she's getting. Why are you attacking her?"

"Because I want to. I don't want her here."

"Why don't you want her here?"

"This is my house and I don't want her interfering with what I'm doing."

"What've you been doing?"

"I don't have to tell you."

"Okay I'll tell you - you've been playing with her emotions. Every time she feels happy you give her sad feelings, and when she's down you push her feelings further down."

"So what are you going to do about it?"

"Offer you the chance to go to heaven and be with your family. If you don't want to do that, we will have to remove you from this house and place you in a bubble of calming energy while our guides have a chat with you and try to help you to understand your situation."

"First, I'm not going anywhere and I certainly don't want to be with my family, and second, I would just come back when you've gone."

I was aware there were two others working with him.

"If you could've got out of the protection we've put round the house, you wouldn't be here now. Once we place you and your two friends in the bubble of light, you will not be able to come back."

"Do what you like. We'll see what happens."

"You and your two friends can go and speak to our guides - my advice is to listen to what is said to you."

Once she had made sure they were gone, the trance medium – Carol - came back and said:

"He wasn't very pleased with you, I had a job holding back what he was calling you, and I watched them go - they weren't very happy."

"Yes, he was trying to get away from his boss, who wasn't pleased they'd been caught."

Rose said: "Can I ask a question?"

"Yes of course," I said.

"How did you know where they were and how did you get them to come through?"

"When I went round the house I could feel them. As I go round, I sense who are good and who aren't. I then work on getting the worst through first and dealing with them. That gives the lost souls a sense of relief and a feeling of safety. They're more willing to come and talk to us, without fear of repercussions from the nasty ones, because we've already removed them. It's as though I'm putting them in order, so that I know who to get through first. I usually start with the obvious ones, who are the least experienced and then work my way up to the person in charge. Once I've detected where they are, I then ask the trance medium to tune in to them by giving part of a description. When they have the right person, they then give me a bit more about them. In that way I know they have the right one. Although they don't want to come through, we're able to encourage them to come and talk to us with the help of our guides, while we determine how best to help them and you. When we've sorted out their situation, we then either help them if they are lost, or - like those three - we remove them."

"How did you know there was more than one?"

"I'm fed information from my guides while I'm talking to them. That's why it's so important to know who your guides are. We work as a team - that's how I knew what he and his friends had been doing. Some of the spirits we talk to are more forthcoming but some will tell lies, as you'll see as we progress."

"How do you remove them, and what's a bubble?"

"We work very closely with our guides and with their help the bad spirits are removed. The bubble is an energy that restricts them from doing things to you or anyone else. It takes a long time for them to come to terms with what they have been doing sometimes. During that time, our guides and their relatives try to help them understand what they have been doing is wrong. They also help them to accept they now belong in the light. Eventually they all move into the light to continue their spiritual journey. The only way you'll have any more problems when we've finished is if you invite others in. By that I mean that there are others who will take over from them. What's been going on is in your aura, and if different spirits come in they'll read that and carry on with it. That way you'll think this hasn't worked. By doing it that way it's easier for them, as they're using what has already worked - it will also make you think you're stuck with them."

"I don't want them back."

"I know, but sometimes if you've had the problem for a while, it becomes normal to you, and you may instinctively invite others in by mistake. Don't worry, we'll monitor the situation, and deal with any problems if they arise. We'll carry on with the rest of them now, as there are some more to clear and a lot to help."

"Do you mean there are more of them?" Rose asked.

"Yes, it takes quite a lot of them to do all the different things that you've been experiencing, but don't worry - we'll remove them all. You see, it's like your house has been taken over by nasty spirits, and they either don't want you here, or are using you to practise on and control."

"Why do they do it?"

"Where they are, they have nothing else to do, and they find they have this ability to influence you, to mess around with your emotions and feelings without, most of the time, getting caught. There aren't many people who will get involved in clearing them, so they mostly have free reign over what they do, and who they do it to. What they do is take over a house or building and bring in spirits that are lost, on the pretext that they're helping them. Once they're caught, they can't - or don't know how to - get away, so they're at the mercy of their captors. They then show these lost spirits how to mess around with your feelings, so they can control you. Although the lost souls don't want to upset you, they're made to do it. If they don't do as they're told, they'll get the same thing done to them. Some of the earthbound spirits are suffering from pains or ailments or are just depressed, and by making them come into your aura, the pain or discomfort they feel is picked up by you. They're ruled by fear; that's how they keep them under control. Let me give you an example: the nasty spirits are able to control lost souls because they can put thoughts into their minds of things that will frighten them, as they can do to you. They manipulate the thought process and make them think it's really happening, just as they do to you. It's like when you dream - it's really happening to you, isn't it? Over there, the lost spirits don't know where or how to get help. If they knew all they had to do was ask, then this kind of thing wouldn't be happening."

"Why don't the lost spirits go to heaven? I thought everyone did."

"The problem is there are a lot of people who don't realise they've died, for lots of reasons - maybe there was a sudden accident. Sometimes things happen in hospital that weren't expected and people die, and suddenly they're in a different place. There are many that believe there's nothing after this life, so imagine their surprise when things seem to be carrying on, but in a different way. If you've believed there was nothing, or you just go to sleep, imagine what you must feel when you die and find there's more. Then there are those who have been misguided by religion into believing that someone - Jesus - will come and meet them, and he doesn't. They usually think they're bad or have sinned, so have to work through some kind of penance before they can be taken to heaven. Just think if you were a nun who had dedicated your life to God, and believed Jesus would be waiting for you when you died, how would you feel knowing you had passed and he wasn't there to meet you? Pretty confused, don't you think? So it's not only those people who have died in sudden or unusual ways that get lost, there are many who - through their beliefs - are lost."

"But I thought everyone had a guardian angel looking after them."

"That's true in a way. We all have many guides who work with us all through our lives, who are in the spirit realms. They are not allowed to force themselves on us when we pass, because of free will. It's like they say: 'ask and you will receive'. If you don't know you can ask, or who to ask, then you won't, will you? I'm sure you've heard of people who saw a tunnel with a light at the end in near-death experiences. Or others whose relatives, who had already passed, came to visit them when their time was near. These are not hallucinations or fantasies - it really is happening. You see, your loved ones do come to greet you, and help you to prepare for the next world. Unfortunately when people pass suddenly, unless they're aware of the spirit world or their guides, their loved ones don't get the chance to prepare them."

"What about your guides? Why can't you see them when you die?"

"You have to remember you've just spent a lifetime in the physical body and you're used to how it works. Think how you would feel without it, providing you noticed it was gone. Because you're so used to the body, there's nothing initially to make you think you don't still have it, unless you know you've died. You will still - even then - see with your eyes, because that's how you always have, but you will only see the physical world. It's not an easy concept to get your head round: spirit, which is now you, not only doesn't have a body, but doesn't see in the way you're used to. While wandering around in the spirit realms close to the earth, you will still be able to see the people on the earth plane. But they won't see you, unless they're mediumistic or very sensitive. Spirit see with their senses and this is why most lost souls can't see their guides; they're still looking with their eyes. Most mediums have to learn to open their senses to receive information from spirit. Those who work in the spirit realms, on the nasty side, know where these lost souls are and choose to work around the earth plane, in the hopes of either communicating with people or just manipulating them. They know about heaven - in fact some of them have been there but choose to leave, as they consider it more fun to upset people like you. They don't have the opportunity to be guides and work with us on the earth plane, but they seem to want to stay around us. Sometimes they're trying to get revenge for the things they've suffered while they were here, and sometimes they're just plain nasty. The fact that you don't know them, and haven't done anything to them, makes no difference. They just want to get their own back by striking out, like a child, at the nearest person. Then there are those who want power - usually they were either used to controlling people when they were here, or they've found they can manipulate people on this plane without getting caught. Basically they prey on the innocent, or those that are sensitive, because it's easier. When someone dies in unusual circumstances or gets lost because of what they believe, they're easy prey for these individuals. They promise to help them, then turn on them and force them to do things to people here."

"What do they get out of it apart from revenge? There's no money in spirit, is there? They must be doing it for other reasons."

"It's all about power. They will take over houses and offices in this world and use them as training areas. They can then train those they capture, and trade them with each other, to gain other abilities they don't have themselves. In this way they build up a large inventory of abilities. This makes it easier for them to interfere with us, and also defend themselves against others like themselves who want to take away their properties. They will also attack each other; if they succeed they will own another property, which gives them more power. Does that make things clearer?"

"Yes, a little. I would never have thought they would be so busy interfering with us."

"They've got nothing else to do. Shall we continue with the spirits in your house? There's a woman with long black hair, about five four, slim build, her hair is a bit straggly, Can you tune in to her?"

One of the sitters said: "Has she got a man, about fortyish, standing next to her?"

"Yes, that's her. Will you bring her through please?"

The sitter brought her through.

"What have you been doing here?" I said.

"I haven't been doing anything - just watching what's been going on."

"So why are you here?"

"I was sent here to look after the children."

"When you say look after the children, don't you mean make sure they do as they're told?"

"Yes of course. Can't have them doing nothing, can we?"

"So what have you been making them do?"

"Oh, they just move things around and hide things."

Rose said: "That's why I keep losing things."

"So you're making them move things to annoy the lady who lives here?"

"It's just a bit of fun - there's nothing else to do."

"Have you considered how that might upset the lady?"

"She'll get used to it. It's not doing any harm."

"That's not the point. Not only are you making her think she may be going mad, but you shouldn't be here either."

"Who are you to tell me I shouldn't be here? I'm not doing any harm. Anyway, she isn't complaining."

"Rose, tell her how you feel about that."

"I don't want you here disrupting my life and messing about with my things. I want you to leave," Rose said.

"Well," I said. "She can't put it any clearer than that, can she? Rose wants you out of her house. Would you and your friend like to go to heaven and meet your loved ones?"

"We've looked for heaven but couldn't find it, so we decided this was all there was. Can you take us to heaven?"

"Yes, if you want to go, we would be happy to."

"If there really is a heaven we'd both like to go, if they'll have us. We've not been very nice to the children."

"The children will be fine - we're going to take them all to heaven in a minute. We'll help you first. Can you open your eyes and tell me what you can see?"

"I can see a tunnel with a light at the end."

"That's the entrance to heaven where we're going to take you."

"But why couldn't we see that before?"

"Because you were looking with your eyes. Now you're in the spirit realms you have no eyes - you have to use your senses. By asking you to open your eyes, we've enabled you to automatically open your senses. That's why you can see where you are now."

"Can we go to heaven now?"

"Yes if you would like to. Come with me. I'll take you to your loved ones."

When we arrived in the light, they could see their parents and the rest of their families who had gone over before them. I asked:

"Do you want to stay here with your families and friends?"

"Yes please and thank you for your help. We're sorry for upsetting the lady."

"Well, all's well that ends well. Goodbye."

"Goodbye, and thanks again."

The sitter opened his eyes and said: "I watched them go but they left a lot of children behind."

" "We'll sort them out in a minute. I just want to get rid of the nasty spirits. The children will feel safer when they're gone. There's a brother and sister trying to hide in the bathroom. Can anyone tune in to them?" I said

"Yes, I've got the man - he's not very nice at all."

"Have you got a tall thin man with a big nose and black hair combed straight back?"

"Yes that's him and he's trying to hide behind the woman."

"Will you bring him through please?"

As he came through, Rose looked a bit uncomfortable.

"Are you feeling alright?"

"No, I'm getting a terrible headache."

" Just hang on - I'll deal with that first." I said to the man: "You can tell your sister to stop what she's doing to Rose, or we'll have to block her, which won't be very nice for her." After a moment I said to Rose: "How are you feeling now?"

Rose said: "It's going now - that's much better, thanks."

"Why were you trying to hide behind your sister? A bit cowardly, don't you think? You should know by now you can't hide or leave until we've had a little chat."

"It was worth a try. Anyway, you've no business here - this is our house. Why don't you mind your own business?"

"I have every right to be here, as I was invited by the lady that lives here. As you've probably gathered, we're here to try and help people like you and your sister."

"You're going to have to be a lot tougher than you are to get rid of us - we've been here a long time, and we're staying."

"Really? Then how come, if we're not tough enough, you're here talking to me, especially when you tried to hide? If you're so tough, what were you frightened of?"

"I'm not frightened of anything - it was just tactics to see how good you are."

"Well now you know. Why have you and your sister been playing with the lady's emotions? What do you get out of upsetting her?"

"We want the house to ourselves so we can get on with our business without interference from her."

"How is she interfering with you? You're the one who's attacking her."

"Every time we get things how we want it, she fights back and causes disruption among the kids. We have to sort them out before we can get on with their training."

"I'm afraid you can't stay here - we're clearing this house of all your associates and taking the lost souls to heaven, where they will be safe."

"You'll have a job. You have got to get rid of me and my sister first."

"You can either let us take you to heaven, or be placed in a bubble of light while our guides and your families talk to you. It's your choice."

"I'm certainly not going to heaven - it's full of pansies. I'll leave by myself with my sister."

"If heaven were full of pansies, where do you think our guides come from? As for leaving of your own accord with your sister, be my guest, but you'll both be placed in separate bubbles. You're free to go now: say goodbye to your sister."

Our guides took them away and we could feel the difference in the energy in the house; it was much calmer.

"I am aware of a number of children in the house. I think we should help them now."

"Can I ask a question?" Rose said.

"Yes of course. How are you feeling now?"

"Much better thanks. I didn't realise there were so many. Why are there children here?

"The children are gathered up when they get lost and brought here - they're then made to do things. If they have a pain, they're made to merge their aura with yours - in that way you can feel their pain as if it were yours. They are also taught how to affect your emotions. If they don't do as they're told, they get into a lot of trouble. They're so frightened they will do anything just to be left alone."

"Where do they get the children from? I thought the innocent would go straight to heaven."

"There are lots of reasons why children and adults don't go straight to heaven, as I was saying earlier. When a child dies in traumatic circumstances, sometimes they don't even know they've died. It doesn't happen to all of them, but if you consider how many children have died that way over, say, the last 50 years all over the world, and if only one percent gets lost, that's an awful lot of children who need help. Some may have been taught that their god or representative will meet them when they die, so they'll wait until they're met. When no-one meets them, they're confused. Let's face it - how many times have you seen a child's face when they're told something by an adult? They don't question it, because they're taught that adults know what they're talking about. They wouldn't question the local vicar or priest because they're told he works for God and knows what he's talking about. It's the same with any religion. The religious leaders indoctrinate the parents and the children grow up following their parents' beliefs. Why shouldn't they? They don't know any different. There are many situations where children die in frightening circumstances and their fear is still with them when they get to the other side. The children then get lost in the spirit realms, and are easy prey for the likes of those we've just been dealing with. It's not just children - there are plenty of adults in the same situation."

I asked if there were any more questions at the moment and when Rose said 'no', I said:

"Let's sort out the children and the adults who have been brought here."

I asked the trance mediums, of which there were two, to tune in and tell me what they were picking up. Immediately one of the mediums said:

"I'm picking up a young girl who's standing over there with her brother."

"Tell us about her, please," I said

"She's about six years old and has fair hair about shoulder length and her brother is about two years older."

" I've got them. Would you like to bring the brother through please?"

The little boy came through and it was plain to see he was very nervous.

"Hello, Timothy, how are you?"

"I'm a bit frightened. Who are you?"

"My name is Mike - we've come to help you. We know you've been lost, and those horrible people have been making you do things to the lady, but they're gone now."

"So they can't get me anymore, or my sister?"

"No we've removed them and they can't come back. You're safe now."

"My sister's very frightened too."

"I know, but everything will be alright now. Do you know what's happened to you?"

"Sort of - we aren't the same as we were, and it's dark and cold here. There were a lot of horrible people making us do nasty things to the lady. I'm sorry, we didn't want to, but they made us."

"Yes we know. Tell me the last thing you remember before it got dark and cold."

"We were at home and mummy's new boyfriend came in drunk, and he hit mummy and then tried to hit my sister. She got out of the way and he missed and fell over. I grabbed her hand

and we ran and hid in the bedroom, then we heard him come in and he was shouting. We were very frightened - he hadn't been as bad as that before."

"What happened next?"

"He started looking for us, but we were hiding under the bed - we thought he couldn't see us, but he did. Then he pulled my sister out and started hitting her and she fell over and just lay there. I crept out the other side of the bed as he was bending over to hit her again and kicked him as hard as I could."

"I know this is not easy, but it will help you in a minute."

"It was very frightening. He grabbed me and threw me against the wall and I banged my head. Then it all went dark."

"What happened next?"

"I don't know - we were just in the dark and a women came up to us and said, 'come with me and I'll look after you'."

"When your head gets banged on the wall as hard as that and it goes dark, what do you think would happen to you?"

"I don't know. I suppose if you hit your head that hard it would break."

"If your head breaks, what does that mean?"

"I think it would mean I'm dead, but I'm standing up talking to you. You can't do that if your dead, can you?"

"Where do you go when you die, do you know?"

"Mummy says Jesus comes and gets you and takes you to heaven."

"Well you do go to heaven, but Jesus won't be coming to get you."

"If I've died, this must be heaven then. It's not very nice and there are lots of people who're horrible here."

"No, you haven't gone to heaven yet because you got lost, but we're going to take you there to see your granny."

"How do you know my granny's in heaven? Do you know her?"

"No, but while I've been talking to you, I've been looking for her. I've found her now. She's not very big but she wears an apron with a pocket in the front full of sweets. She says these are for my precious little children."

With a smile Timothy said: "That's my granny - she always had some sweets for us and she used to call us her precious children."

"Would you and your sister like to go and stay with her?"

"Yes please. Does she know we're here?"

"Yes and she's waiting for you because I told her we'd found you. Now, Timothy, will you help me to take all the other children who're there with you, to see their families too?"

"There are a lot here - yes I will."

"Alright let's get all the children together. Open your eyes and tell me what you can see."

"I can see a tunnel with a big light at the end."

"Yes that light's in heaven and the tunnel is how we're going to go there. Can you see the shiny people?"

"Yes, who are they? They're all around us making sure we keep together, like our teachers did, when we went somewhere from school."

"They're our friends and they're making sure we don't lose anyone. Now does your head still hurt?"

"Yes a little."

"We'll take away the pain and make everyone better now. How does that feel?"

"My head doesn't hurt anymore and my sister says she feels alright too."

"Good - is everyone ready?"

"Yes, we're all ready."

"Off we go. It won't take long. It's nice and warm now, isn't it?"

"Yes and I can see people."

"Let's get a little closer. Now do you recognise anyone?"

"Yes I can see my granny and granddad is with her too."

"Would you like to stay with them?"

"Yes please. I can see all the other children going to their families too."

"Good - off you go then. You'll be safe now."

"Thank you, mister." And they were gone.

I looked at Rose and saw there were tears running down her face. I asked her:

"Are you alright?"

"Yes, I'm just sad that those little children were killed like that and have had to suffer so much."

"The children have been living in the 'now', so it's like it all happened a minute ago. Although they've been through so much, they're not aware of the passage of time, and they're alright now. We have a lady over there - who would like to bring her through?"

"I will," said June, another of the trance mediums.

June brought the lady through and I asked her what her name was.

"I'm Ethel. Where have the children gone?"

"Hello, Ethel. We've taken them to heaven. Are you alright?"

"I'm alright. Are the children safe now?"

"Yes, now we want to help you. Thank you for trying to look after the children - it must have been difficult."

"There were some nasty people here, but they seem to have gone too. They were making the children do all sorts of things to her."

"What were they making the children do?"

"They would get about ten of them and teach them how to play with her emotions. Then they made them attack her all at once - the children were so scared of what they would do to them if they didn't, so they attacked her."

"What were they made to do?"

"Well, when she was happy they made her sad, and then they would give her a feeling of being unwell, and they just had to keep doing it until they had driven her into a depression. Then the children were made to change tactics and make her feel tired: when she went to bed they would make her feel wide awake or they would get into her mind and give her horrible thoughts. In that way they could give her bad dreams. That's how they kept at her, until she didn't know whether she was coming or going."

"Why did they leave you alone? Didn't they make you do things too?"

"Yes, they made me make her angry with her partner and after a while he got fed up and left. The idea was to isolate her, and keep her for themselves so they could practise on her."

"What were they practising for?"

"To teach the children, so they could swap them with others like themselves to get even more ... well, I can only call them slaves, as that's how they were treated."

"I see well they're safe now. Would you like to get away from here?"

"Yes, but where would I go? If I go out there someone else will catch me?"

"No, we can take you to heaven if you want and you can be with Bert."

"Can you really take me to my husband - is he in heaven?"

"Yes, if you open your eyes and tell me what you can see."

"I can see a long tunnel with a bright light at the far end."

"That light is the entrance to heaven. Would you like to go there?"

"Yes please. What about the other people here? They're not bad - can they come as well?"

"Of course they can. I was just going to ask if you would help us to take them with us. Are you in any pain?"

"No, but some of the others are."

"We will take the pain away now. There - is that better?"

"Yes, they're smiling now and nodding, so they must be alright."

"Let's go into the tunnel. There - it's much warmer now, isn't it? We'll be in the light in a moment."

"Yes and I can see people over there."

"Can you see Bert?"

"Yes and I can see my parents. Is it alright if I go and join them?"

"Yes, go in peace."

"God bless you and thank you from all of us. Goodbye."

June came back and I checked the house out again: apart from a small boy hiding, there was no-one else. I came back into the room and asked Carol to tune in to the boy and bring him through.

"Hello. There's no need to be frightened now - the nasty people have gone."

"Are you sure? They were doing horrible things to us and I thought you were their friends."

"No, we're not their friends. What's your name?"

"It's James."

"Well, James, do you know where you are and what's happened to you?"

"Yes, the man said I was dead and I had to stay with him - he was going to look after me now. He wasn't too bad at first, but then when we came here he said I had to do things to the lady to make her feel sick. I didn't want to, but he made me hurt all over until I did. I'm sorry if I upset the lady. I didn't want to."

"Well it's over now - he can't hurt you anymore. Where do people go when they die?"

"I was told you go to heaven but I couldn't find it, and nobody would tell me the way."

"That's alright. Would you like us to take you there to stay with your mummy and daddy?"

"Is mummy in heaven? She was alright the last time I saw her. Well, she was upset but she wasn't old or ill or anything."

"How long have you been here, James?"

"I don't know - it seems like yesterday, but it also seems a long time."

"Do you know what year it was when you died?"

"Yes, it was 1963."

"Well its 2000 now, so that was 37 years ago. But don't worry - open your eyes and tell me what you can see."

"I can see a tunnel with a big light in it."

"Yes that's the entrance to heaven. Shall we go into the tunnel?"

"Are you coming too?"

"Yes I'm going to take you there so you don't get lost again on the way. What can you see now?"

"I can see lots of people and mummy is over there. Can I go to her please?"

"Yes, you'll be safe now. Bye."

"Bye."

I knew we had cleared the spirits, both good and bad, from the house but I still felt uneasy. I excused myself and walked round the house again. I was not aware of any spirits but I was picking up some nasty vibes in the lounge. I looked around and felt drawn to a carving of an African head that was displayed on the wall.

"Can I take this off the wall please?" I asked Rose.

"Yes of course - what's wrong?"

As I took the head off the wall, I picked up some nasty feelings coming from it. I asked:

"Where did you get this from, Rose?"

"I got it from a friend - what's wrong with it?"

"There's nothing wrong with it in itself, it's what's been

attached to it."

"What do you mean?"

"Objects absorb vibrations just like anything else. Depending what's been going on around the object, or who's using it, and for what, depends on what it absorbs. Take a house for instance - if there have been happy times, when you walk in you'll feel a light atmosphere around the house. On the other hand if things are sad or bad, then the atmosphere reflects it. You must have been in houses where you've felt uncomfortable." Rose nodded. "That's what I'm talking about. There doesn't have to be anyone in the house - just the unhappy vibration. Have you ever done psychometory?"

"Yes, a couple of times at the church. I know what you mean - that's when you tune in to an object and tell the owner things about it."

"Yes, well this carving is similar to that. Everything has a history and it can be read by picking up its vibrations. With houses, there are usually spirits that are attracted by the misery, or people who are going through bad times. The spirits may even add to the problem, just like you've experienced. But objects can be affected in other ways too. When these things are carved, the person making it may put a chant on it to protect his work. Sometimes the energy that's put into the chant will attract negative spirits, who will then go about the job of protecting the object in question by surrounding it with bad energy. You have to remember the Africans are an ancient civilisation and were very spiritual in the old days. There are many today that believe and invoke spirits to help them in their daily lives. Protecting one's work would be a normal thing for them, especially wood-carvings, as they are made from trees, which are considered by some to be sacred. Occasionally the wrong spirit gets involved and can create unhappy or upsetting atmospheres around the object."

"That's funny - out of all the carvings and things I've collected, I've always felt a bit strange when I look at that one. Shall I throw it away?"

"No, we can remove the bad energies and clear it in a similar way that we've done to the house. We don't look for the spirit that's attached itself - we just ask our guides to clear it. If you like, we'll just give it healing and our guides will do the rest."

"What do they do?"

"If there's a spirit who's attached themselves to it, they'll talk to them. Most of the time the spirit thinks they're helping the person who produced it. They'll help the spirit understand there's no need to protect the object and will deal with them accordingly. Sometimes there are just bad vibrations around the object which have to be neutralised. Either way the object will be cleared as yours is now. Hold it and see what you feel."

"It feels warm - other than that, I can't feel anything."

"That's fine. We don't want you opening up at the moment anyway. It would've made the hairs in the back of your neck stand up if it still had the bad vibes on it."

"I get that happening quite a lot."

"What - the hairs on your neck standing up?"

"Yes. Is that when I'm picking up bad spirits?"

"Usually you will instinctively feel something's wrong, but because you're in your physical body, you tend to ignore it. It's your spirit sensing that something's not right. If you like, you're getting a warning. Some people listen to their instincts, but unfortunately not enough. If they did, there wouldn't be so many problems in this world. That's the last of them - everything's clear now."

"God, I never realised there were so many of them."

"No, most people think there's only one, but as I said earlier, it takes quite a few of the nasty spirits to do things to you."

"How come the children are able to do those things? They're only young."

"You see them as children, but they're experienced spirits and are as capable as the rest of them. They just look like children because they only have that memory of themselves until they get back to heaven. When they cause you discomfort, it's usually the feelings they're having, so just by being close to you they can make you feel what they are feeling. If you weren't so sensitive, you wouldn't feel most of the discomfort they're experiencing. Is there anything else you would like to ask?"

"Yes - you said spirits see with their senses. How do the spirits you help suddenly see the tunnel and the light?"

"When I ask them to open their eyes, their guides help them

to open their senses so they can see the spirit world. They don't realise they can do that, because they usually haven't thought in that way - and why should they? After all they can see, so why should they think they can't?"

"Oh I see."

"Is there anything else?"

"No, I don't think so at the moment."

"Now here's what I want you to be aware of. First, we've cleared your house and there are no nasty spirits left. All the lost souls have been taken to heaven: there are only your guides and loved ones here now. They will not disturb you and you won't be aware of them - they won't move things or make any indication of their presence. Because of the problems you've been experiencing, it will take about two weeks for the vibrations to settle down. In the meantime you must stay closed down and not even look, physically or mentally, to see if there is anyone still here. That's an invitation for others to come in and if they do, they'll copy the things you've been experiencing, to make you think the nasty spirits haven't gone and that we've been wasting our time. Let me reassure you - we have cleared everything out. Now, if you can get on with your life as though nothing like this exists, you should have no more problems. When I say 'stay closed' I mean don't go for healing or to circle for at least two weeks, and don't try and give any clairvoyance. Part of what you're doing is settling down your own mind and the rest is allowing the vibrations to settle down. If you inadvertently open up, then as soon as you're aware that you have, go through your procedure for closing down. I'll leave you my phone number in case you have any problems. Just call any time you need help or advice."

"How do you suggest I close down? I've tried on many occasions and it doesn't seem to work."

"First you must believe it will, then - rather than just saying words - you must visualise yourself closing down and being protected, and ask your guides to assist you. Every time you think you may have opened up, go through the process again."

"Can you suggest the best procedure for me to stay closed and get the best protection?"

"Everyone's different, but I'll give you a run-through of one that I use. Close your eyes and imagine a white ball of light in the pit of your stomach. Then picture it in your mind's eye. Now start to expand it until you're sitting in the middle surrounded in this white light, then ask your guides to help you to maintain it. Once you're satisfied that you're surrounded in light and have asked your guides to help, then believe it and open your eyes. There are a few variations of this procedure and you may have to try some of them until you're comfortable and confident. Whilst you're doing that, you must have the intention in your mind that you will be protected and closed. It's not about the picture or the words - it's the intent that makes the difference. The visualisation only helps you to create the state of mind for it all to work. I'll go through it again, but this time I want you to follow what I say with everything else I have said in mind also."

I talked Rose through it again and at the end she seemed satisfied that she would be able to do it herself.

"How often do I need to do that?" she asked.

"Do it in the morning when you get up and in the evening before you go to bed. If you feel uneasy or are aware of anything during the day, try to find a quiet space for a few moments and do it again. The more you do it, the easier it gets, until in the end you'll be able to close down in a couple of seconds or so."

We talked for a while and as it was getting late, we left.

A Few Days Later

A few days later, in the late afternoon, I got a call from Rose saying she was still having problems. I arranged to go and see her the following morning and this is what transpired. There were two of us, and when we arrived Rose was very apologetic about calling me. I said:

"It's okay, not a problem. Now what's been going on?"

"It was all quiet after you left the other night, but in the morning I started to feel edgy, as if someone was staring at me. Then a bit later I heard all these voices chattering at once in my head. I tried but I couldn't stop it, and I was getting angry, then hyper, then I felt really miserable and depressed."

This could be diagnosed as schizoaffective disorder (mood changes) coupled with residual schizophrenia (feeling miserable and depressed) and paranoid schizophrenia (hearing voices and seeing things and the feeling of being watched). Fortunately we were aware of the spirit interference as soon as we arrived and were able not only to confirm what was happening, but remove the cause.

"Let me check the place out."

I walked round the house and was aware of a number of spirits, so when I got back I asked Rose:

"If you don't mind, I would like you to sit in this chair so that I can give you some healing."

"Do you mean - the same as you did at the church?"

"Yes, you've a number of spirits that have attached themselves to you and I'm going to remove them. Where've you been where it feels uncomfortable?"

"I was round my mum's yesterday - it always has an uncomfortable atmosphere round there. Is that where I got them from?"

"Very likely. I don't suppose you closed down before you went, did you?"

"I was only going round my mum's - I didn't think I would have to."

"That's fair enough, but when you go anywhere in future think about how you felt last time you were there. If you felt in anyway uncomfortable, close down before you go, and when you leave just to be sure."

"Why do I need to close down all the time? Isn't once enough?"

"At the moment, because you're very sensitive, you're a prime target for any nasty spirits that are around. They'll force themselves on you to try to open you up so they can play on your emotions. They've had control of you and they don't want to let go. It's not the spirits we threw out, but there are others who see you as an easy target - at the moment it's a free-for-all to see who can get control of you first. So you must keep checking and closing down. What you're really doing is putting protection around yourself and restating that you don't want these nasty spirits around you. I know it's going to be hard work to start with, but it will become second nature after a while. It's your responsibility to protect yourself and by asking your guides to help, you're showing those in spirit who you want around you and who you don't. Everything that's happened to you is in your aura - those in spirit and some mediums can read that record. That's how they know what's worked before, and they will carry on with the same thing if they can get in. Now we'll get rid of these few who're here now and you'll be clear again, okay?"

"Yes please - I'm sorry to cause so much trouble."

"It's not a problem. Now let's see who we have here."

Once I had extracted those who had attached themselves, I spoke to Carol who had come with me again and said:

"We're going to talk to them now and see if we can help them. There's a little fat man who's wearing a long overcoat and a trilby hat over there. Can you tune in to him?"

"Yes, he's about five foot four and about 40 to 50 years old."

"That's him - if you would bring him through, please."

"Yes."

"Hello. What do you want with this woman?"

"Nothing. I'm just following her around."

"Why are you following her? She would rather be left alone."

"Well I was bored where I was and thought, as she had no one around her, she might get lonely, so I came with her."

"Where did you pick her up? From her mum's house?"

"Yes, it's getting pretty boring there now and I felt like a change."

"Well you can't stay here. What was your intention?"

"I just wanted someone else to work on, you know - try something new."

"So you attached yourself to Rose. Well she doesn't want you, so we're going to give you a choice. You can go to heaven and be with your loved ones or we can place you in a calming bubble of light while you have a conversation with our guides. Which is it to be?"

"I don't want to go to heaven - that's even more boring, I'll just leave then, if she doesn't want my company."

"I'm sorry I can't allow you to just leave, because you'll just attach yourself to someone else. If you don't want to go to heaven then we'll put the bubble of light around you and you can have a chat with our guides. Maybe having a chat will help you to see reason - you'll come to your senses and ask to be taken to heaven."

"What's this bubble and why are you doing this to me? It's none of your business."

"A bubble is an energy that we put round you that will neutralise anything you try to do that may upset others, both in this world and the spirit realms. It'll take a long time for it to wear off, which will hopefully give you time to reconsider your options. The reason we're doing this is because we've been asked to by the lady you've been following, and she's given us the authority to work on her behalf. Now you're free to go and take your five friends with you. You will all be placed in a bubble of light. Goodbye."

Carol came back and said:

"They've all gone now. I was picking up his thoughts - he was going to let you throw him out, and then get his mates to invite him back. He was really annoyed at you when you threw them out as well."

"They try all sorts of tricks, don't they? Now, let's have a word with the woman in the white dress - she has grey hair and wears glasses and is about five foot two in height."

"You mean the slim lady about 60 years old?"

"Yes that's her. Will you bring her through please?" When Carol brought her through, I spoke to her.

106

"Hello - what's your name?"

"My name's Alice. Who are you?"

"My name's Mike and I would like to talk to you."

"What do you want? I don't like to talk to strangers."

"I wanted to know if you're alright."

"No I'm not alright. I have this pain in my chest and my legs hurt and I'm very tired. I haven't slept in a long time and I don't know where I am. I saw this lady and she seemed quite nice, so I thought if I followed her, she might take me to someone who could help me."

"Well she's brought you to us and we'll help you. Let's take the pain away from your legs and chest. There - is that better?"

"Yes. How did you do that?"

"Don't worry. Now we're going to take away that tiredness and then we'll sort out what's happened to you and where you are. Is that better?"

"That's much better, I don't know what you did but if you could bottle it you could sell it."

"Now there's an idea - if only we could! Do you know what's happened to you?"

"Not really. I just seem to have got lost."

"How about if you tell me what you remember and we'll see if we can sort it out."

"I was having my tea when there was a big bang and that's all I can remember."

"Did it go dark?"

"Yes and then I was standing by the table looking down."

"What were you looking at?"

"I thought for a moment I was looking at me, then I realised it couldn't be me, because I was standing up and the person was on the floor."

"I see what else could you see?"

"The whole side of the house had gone and there was a bus in my kitchen."

"So the big bang was a bus crashing through the wall of your kitchen. What do you think may have happened to you if the side of the house collapsed with you in it?"

"I must have been killed - so the person on the floor was me?"

"Yes I'm afraid so. Where do you think people go when they die?"

"Well I suppose it depends, some say there's a heaven and others say there's nothing. There must be something because I'm still here, wherever that is."

"You're right, there is something else. You can go to heaven or you can wander in the dark and cold of the spirit realms. Usually people go to heaven straight away but because you were confused, you got lost. Would you like us to take you to heaven?"

"Yes please - that's why I haven't been sleeping, I thought there was something wrong and there are some horrible people here. I thought you were one of them, which is why I didn't want to talk to you. I've been staying awake so I could hide from them."

"If you'll open your eyes and tell me what you can see?"

"Oh it's very bright - is this heaven?"

"No, but that's where the light's coming from. Your eyes will get used to it in a moment. There are some other people here who're lost - will you help me to take them to heaven too?"

"Yes, it would be a pleasure. They must feel awful too."

"We've taken their pain away. Now, shall we go into the light?"

"Is it far?"

"No, we're there now. What can you see?"

"I can see my husband and he's waving to me. Is it alright if I go to him?"

"Yes of course. Thank you for helping me with the others."

"I didn't do anything, you did it. Thank you for finding me and bringing me home."

"It's our pleasure, go in peace."

"Thank you."

Carol opened her eyes and smiled.

"It was lovely to see her go to her husband. He gave her a big hug."

"It's nice to know we can help, isn't it?"

I looked round at Rose and said:

"They're all gone now. How do you feel?"

"I'm not sure. Am I going to keep getting more of them?"

"Once you've learned to protect yourself, you'll be safe."

"That's what I am worried about - what if I can't protect myself?"

"As I said before, if you believe in what you are doing it will work. Just put the protection around you and ask your guides for help. Don't doubt yourself - it will work, just believe it."

" Thanks for coming round again."

"That's alright. Now don't forget - if you need me, call."

"Alright, but I don't want to bother you."

"It's no bother - you've had a hard time and it'll take a while for you to settle down. Let's just see how things go."

We then left and Rose, though a little unsure, seemed determined to try to hold up her end. On the way home I thought about Rose's situation, and gave some consideration that there might be more to it than meets the eye.

Following up the Second Visit

The following day I telephoned Rose to see how she was getting on and this is what she said:

"Well, I had a bad night, when I looked in the mirror I saw a face. I got very cold and just couldn't close down properly. I got the giggles for no reason and I couldn't stop it. When I went to bed, I tried to close myself down and put protection around myself. I was very tired and as soon as my head hit the pillow I was wide-awake and couldn't settle. Then I heard noises and felt sort of cobwebby round my face, and next thing I know it was 20 minutes later. I felt as though I was in a cocoon - you know, like fine webbing all over me and I couldn't move. After that I felt very low and then a little while later I was hyper. I was getting horrible thoughts about you, and how you were controlling me and I shouldn't let you come here again, and not to talk to you on the phone either. I felt that you were sending me all sorts of thoughts, then I fell asleep."

" How do you feel now?"

"Sort of drained and lethargic. I just can't muster up any enthusiasm to do anything and I've got so much to do."

This is an example of the control spirit can have over someone, yet often it is diagnosed as paranoid schizophrenia, disorganised schizophrenia and schizoaffective disorder, but really it is just spirit interference.

"It sounds like they're getting more intense and, as I suspected, we're going to have a fight on our hands."

"I don't want to waste your time - you must have other things to do. I think I must be going mad."

"No you're not - they're just trying to isolate you so they can have you all to themselves. If they can make you think you're going mad, then they think I will leave you to get on with it, but remember what I said - I'm here for you 24/7. If it's convenient, I'll come over and we'll sort it out."

"Well if you're sure ... thanks for listening to me. Do you really think it's spirit and not me going off my head?"

"I know it's not you because I've come across this sort of thing before, and when I was there yesterday and things were happening, I could feel spirit around you before you noticed anything."

When I arrived I could see she hadn't had a good night: there was that haunted look in her eyes again. She looked at me warily. I was aware there was a heavy presence of nasty spirits and closed myself down. I sat in the armchair, after Rose sat on a chair - she was perched right on the edge, not at ease at all. I asked her to tell me what had been happening. Rose said:

"I feel very vulnerable at the moment. It's as though someone is sitting in my lap."

"Shall we start by closing you down and then we'll sort out the rest of it,?"

"Yes, alright."

I went through the process with Rose and while she was doing that, I gave her healing to help settle her down. Once she had closed down, we talked about what had been happening.

"I think the first thing we need to do is stop the chatter in your mind," I said. "Then we can move on to the rest of it. I want you to do a meditation which I will talk you through. First, take my hands and close your eyes. Now picture in your mind a brick wall all around you."

" I'm trying to picture a brick wall, but it keeps falling down and I'm aware of a presence behind me."

"Right - open your eyes and look at me. Now picture in your mind a brick wall that goes up and up until it's out of sight. The wall is ten feet thick and very old. Keep looking at me. When you can see the wall, notice it's in front of you and goes all the way round you. The only way in is through your mind - there is no door and it's so high no-one can get in over the top. Believe what I tell you and you'll find that, if you concentrate on the wall in front of you, the chatter will gradually fade out as you concentrate more. They're playing mind games with you, and now you're giving them some of their own medicine. Believe in yourself and your guides and ask them to maintain the wall. Is that better?"

"Yes, the chatter is fading but it hasn't gone. It's like I've had people in my head for years and suddenly it's not as bad."

"Yes and with practice you will get things under your control. The fact that the chatter has faded is a measure of the strength of your mind."

We stopped the meditation and as I watched I could feel a cold draft swirling around Rose. Her face became like plaster, very pale, and she started giggling. She was being possessed. I took her hand and told her to hang on and said to the spirit:

"What do you want with her?"

The voice was Rose's, but somehow more masculine, and it said:

"We want her, and all the time you're around her we'll be working on you and we'll get you."

I smiled and said:

"It's been tried in the past. Leave her alone - she doesn't want you around."

As I was saying this, I asked my guides to remove the spirit and place him in a bubble so that he couldn't come back. Rose's face cleared and she was back in this world and very upset.

"It happened again, didn't it? I know I was giggling but I couldn't stop. What's going on?"

"You're being taken over by nasty spirits and we've just got rid of that one. How often does this happen?"

"It happens quite often, especially when I'm feeling low. I seem to go a bit hyper, then I get depressed, then that happens and I can't stop it. It happens before I realise, and by then it's too late."

This could be diagnosed as split personality disorder or bipolar, where in actual fact it's spirit again, interfering with Rose's thoughts and taking over her mind for a short period.

"Well now you have me to watch over you and I'll let you know when it's coming, so we can get it under control. What you need to do is stay calm at all times. When you're aware you're getting low, do something to change you energy, even if it's just walking round the room or putting on some music. Staying calm is the trick - if you can keep your emotions level not too happy, and not too sad, then it will be harder for them to get at you, and you'll remain in control of your feelings. It won't happen straight away - we'll need to work at it - but I'll let you know when your mood changes and we can monitor it. As far as the face in the mirror is concerned, you have to ignore it. Don't let it frighten you and try to keep your emotions the same. "

"This is going to be very hard. How will I know if it's me and not spirit?"

"It doesn't matter - try to keep calm anyway, then you won't give them an opening. They're going to be with you for a while trying to get to you, and the protection will only work for a while. As I said before, they will work at it until they find a way in, so you need to give them as little chance as possible. With practice you'll be able to ignore them and as your strength builds they'll affect you less. The most important thing is to stay on an even keel with your emotions."

"I'm fed up with being controlled by them. I will not be beaten - with your help we will win."

"That's the spirit! With that kind of attitude you'll soon see the difference and have more control over your life. But don't forget, you'll bounce backwards and forwards for a while as you start to get things under control."

I stayed at Rose's for the rest of the day and when it was time for me to leave she seemed very apprehensive. I asked her what was troubling her and she said:

"I'm worried that as soon as you go I'll get attacked and I won't be able to stop it."

"What you must remember is fear breeds fear. If you're frightened something is going to happen, it's almost as if you're inviting it. Try to forget about them. I know it's not going to be easy, but if you can focus on what you're doing, it will make it harder for them."

As I was about to go, I felt a cold feeling all down my back and a prickly feeling around my head. I looked at Rose and saw her eyes start to change. I took her hands in mine and led her to the sofa and sat her down. As I did so, she started singing nursery rhymes. I spoke to her but got no response, so I held her hands and created a bubble of energy around us both and gently talked to her until she started to take notice. The look in her eyes changed and she was back with me. Rose was very upset.

"Something just happened, didn't it? I must be a nut job. I don't even have control of my own mind."

"Did you feel it go very cold just as I was about to leave?"

"Yes, but I thought it was just a breeze when you opened the door."

"No, that was spirit coming close. You're not nuts - I felt things changing before it even affected you."

"Can't you stop it?"

"No, I can teach you how to, but it has to come from you. Your protection is not being set up properly - tell me what you're doing."

I left Rose to compose herself and while she was doing that, I made her a cup of tea. When she was settled, I asked again for her to run through what she did when she was closing down and protecting herself.

"Well first I imagine a flower open, then I close it and try to picture a white light. I then try to expand it so it covers me completely and ask my guides to help and protect me. I have trouble picturing the flower and sometimes I see a sort of cocoon all round me. I can't seem to get rid of it, then the white light keeps disappearing and I just end up hoping it's there and that I've done it properly."

"We'll have to change what you're doing a bit, because it's not doing the job. Probably because you're not able to get things in focus. Let's try again to get you closed down."

"It's so hard - are you sure it's the only thing you can do?"

"There are many things we can do, but we have to get this right first. Now, I'll hold your hands and I want you to close your eyes. Now regulate your breathing until it's comfortable, because at the moment you're breathing much too fast. As you concentrate on your breathing, allow yourself to become calm and peaceful. We'll do that for a while until you settle, and while you are doing that I'll give you some healing to help settle you down."

"Why is it so easy for them to take me off?"

"Partly because you're so sensitive, and partly because they've been doing it for a long time, so it's easy to get into you. Also because it's been happening for a long time, you half expect it. It's not your fault - they've got you conditioned so you're receptive to them. It's been a major part of your life for so long and we have to change your expectations and beliefs. Now that you're settled, I want you to picture your flower open and watch the petals closing."

"I can't seem to picture the flower and I feel kind of wobbly."

"Go back to your breathing and open your eyes for a while until you're feeling more settled. Now, see that flower over there? I want you to stare at it and get a good picture in your mind's eye.

Now while you're staring, close your eyes but still see the flower. Have you still got it?"

"Yes, it's still there."

"Good. Now I'm going to tune in to your flower as well and together we'll close the petals. See them slowly closing and think to yourself that you're closing down. Believe you're closing yourself down - don't forget you can do this all day, but if you don't believe it you're wasting your time. Now this time we're going to picture a column of light above your head. We're going to allow it to come down through your crown chakra and then on through the rest of your chakras until you're completely engulfed in the light. Can you see that?"

"Yes, it's quite clear at the moment."

"Good. Now you should be thinking that the light is your protection - ask your guides to help and protect you. Have you done that?"

"I'm waiting to see my guides come and take over."

"You won't see your guides unless you open up again and the object of this exercise is to close down. Your guides can hear you. You don't have to see them, just trust that they're there. When you've done that, open your eyes."

"That's done - now what?"

"Your protection is only part of what you have to do. Now you have to ignore anything that's not normal, or a change in thought or attitude. You still have to protect yourself - your guides are allowed to do so much and you have to do the rest. If you like, you have to show your intentions all the time by rejecting any approach by nasty spirits. I know it's difficult at the moment, but you have to keep asserting your will to overcome the negativity they keep throwing at you. You'll win some and lose some, but gradually over time, you will win. You just have to keep at it."

"But I'm getting so tired of having to keep fighting. When's it all going to end?"

"It will get easier, but will never end. You will just be in control and your mind will be strong enough to overcome the feelings they give you. Now I know you're still unsure of yourself, so if you like, I'll stay for a while and watch over you."

"I can't take up any more of your time - you must have other things to do. I'll be alright. Maybe I'm a bit off my head."

"Actually you're not. I felt the nasty spirits attacking you earlier and I'm aware of them round us now. You just have to focus on what you're doing and ignore what's going on around you spiritually."

"If they're around us now, does that mean they're going to attack me again?"

"They're around you all the time, it just depends on how focussed you are on what you're doing as to how easy it is for them to get to you. Even your protection will hold them for a short while, but you have to back it up with your own control. Try to keep your emotions level at all times - don't get angry or too happy, just stay cool and it will be much more difficult to get in."

"What if I don't notice the change? They will get me then, won't they?"

"Yes, but each time they get you, you'll learn something new about how they do it. You'll build up your protection as you gain more insight into what they're doing to you."

We talked a little more and once I was satisfied that Rose was feeling more confident, I left.

The Following Week

I didn't hear from Rose for a few days, but when she telephoned and told me what was happening, I felt things weren't going as well as they might. I asked Rose how she was doing.

"I woke up a few times during the night," she said, "and I had the feeling it was another form of attack - am I right?"

"Yes, they're going to try all sorts of things to get at you. The most vulnerable time for anyone is when you're just dozing off and when you're just waking up. This is because you're neither in this world nor the spirit world. As you probably know, when we go to sleep we leave our bodies and go into the spirit world, mostly to have a chat with our guides to make sure we're on the right track. Some people will go and work in the spirit world while they're asleep."

"I tried to close down the first two times and thought I'd succeeded. The third time I was woken, I believe I saw and felt my flower being forced open. That got me annoyed and I tried extra hard and did close down and put myself and my flower in the white light. Do you believe me? Is this real? Did this happen?"

"Yes, I believe you and yes, it did happen. What you were experiencing was the nasty spirits trying to sow self- doubt. If they can persuade you that it doesn't work, then you're back to square one. They'll play with your emotions and try to make you think you can't protect yourself, but believe me you are. If you hadn't, there would have been no point in trying to make you think the flower wasn't working, would there?"

"No, I suppose not. When I woke up I was feeling very depressed, I think because I thought I'd failed."

"Well you certainly didn't fail, because you managed to close down twice when you were woken. The fact that you had trouble the third time shows you how successful you were, since they attacked you even more forcibly the third time."

"I still woke up feeling depressed and the last time I felt that way was over ten years ago. I was also given a vision, and felt the emotions of why I felt that way so long ago. Why would I be remembering these things?"

"Everything that you've experienced is in your aura. It's no big deal for spirit to bring to the forefront of your mind - whatever situation will help them get at you. We're all vulnerable at times -

it's just how we are. The test is to overcome our vulnerabilities and move on. But the memories are still there in your subconscious. You've overcome them before so you can do it again, even when they're enhanced by spirit."

"I've managed to overcome the obstacle, and feel much better having spoken to you. Is this part of the process? Is my strength being tested?"

"Yes, it is part of the process and you'll go backwards and forwards as you get stronger. But as you get stronger so will they - you see, you'll overcome the weaker ones and you'll get stronger and more subtle attacks as you progress. Because you're so sensitive you'll at times find it hard to cope, but don't give up, because you are winning, and you'll know that by how the attacks change."

"When you say the attacks will change, what do you mean?"

"I mean they'll get more subtle and you'll wonder whether it's your thoughts or not. Their idea is to make you think it's all in your mind. Just remember, if you get a sudden change in thought or feelings, then there is a good chance it's not you."

"To be honest, I just wanted to run away this morning, but that would have been cowardly and immature. I realised I needed help and guidance and that you were the only one who has understood the things that have been happening to me. Thank you for your help. Now I know I'm not mad and there is a light at the end of the tunnel. Many challenges were given to me this afternoon that I had to deal with differently. I'm happy with the results - small steps. I've found my senses have become more acute, as noises and smells are clearer than ever. However, a stumbling block of how to deal with the negative energies that I pick up from people has become one of my greatest challenges, and no doubt my strength will be tested."

"Yes, you'll find things becoming more obvious to start with as they step up the attacks. They're just trying to beat you into thinking there's nothing you can do to stop it - they've become a little blasé about things. Because you're so sensitive and they're so clumsy, things will come thick and fast to start with. But as you deal with each attack, they will become more subtle. The reason for that is the more they can make you think it's your own mind, the more chance that you will accept it and give in. Whatever you do, don't go down that route - you're right in your thoughts, so stick with them. If you have any doubts, call me and we'll talk it through and see what is you and what isn't. They work on many different levels of abilities - those who have just learnt are still pretty clumsy in their approach and attacks. As you overcome them, there will be others standing in line that are more skilled at manipulating your feeling and emotions. They're much more subtle, and their objective is to try and get you back to thinking it's your mind. They don't let go easily once they've got you, and they're particularly annoyed at the moment because, up until now, you've been putty in their hands. Now you're getting some guidance and understanding of what they've been and are doing to you, and you're more aware of what is and isn't you. Therefore you're becoming stronger and more capable of defending yourself, but don't think this is going to be easy or over quickly - it will take time. You've been under their control for a long time, and it will take a while to defeat them. You're doing very well and as long as you stick to what you're doing, then we will win."

"I was talking to my mum this morning and she was telling me she used to play with the Ouija board when she was younger. Her house is very cold and in the flat we used to live in before that, there were a lot of noises and things being moved. Were these negative spirits making those noises and things?"

"Yes, very probably. The thing is, when you play with things like the Ouija board then it's like picking up the telephone and dialling a number - any number - and getting an answer. You don't know who is answering and what sort of person it is. Well, when you play with the Ouija board it's the same thing - you don't know what sort of spirit's coming through. It's an invitation and a lot of the time they'll take it that you asked them to come. They will then stay and try to communicate in all sorts of ways, as they consider it's their opportunity to work with someone on the earth plane. Time means nothing to them and they can, and will, follow people to whom they have attached themselves all the way through their lives, unless the person is strong enough to ignore or get rid of them. Often people who hear negative voices in their head or around them are being plagued by this sort of spirit."

"That makes a lot of sense when you put it like that. Have they followed me here, since I also had a go at the Ouija board once, but it wasn't in this house?"

"There can be many reasons for you to be having problems, but I would say there's an even chance that because you're so sensitive, coupled with what you've experienced when living at home with your mum and what you've both been up to with the Ouija board, that you've attracted negative spirits to you."

"So I'm to blame for all this happening to me, then?"

"No, you've been brought up in an environment that appears to have negative spirits around for most, if not all, of your life. For you it became the normal way of things. Because you're sensitive, it's been easier for them to affect you and your life. That's why it'll take time and effort to get rid of them - they're so entrenched in your mind that they'll take some shifting. The problem is because it's been 'normal' to you, we have to re-educate you as to what really is normal to most people."

"Will I ever be able to get rid of them and lead a normal life?"

"Yes of course - we just have to work at it until they're defeated."

"Thanks for talking to me. I'll keep at it. Sometimes it's very hard to tell what is and isn't me, though."

"When you get in that situation, call me and we'll talk it through. In fact, call me if you have any questions or problems. Alright?"

"Yes – thanks. See you soon. Bye."

"Bye and don't forget what I've said."

"I will."

It was interesting to see how Rose was coping with her problems compared to how she had been a week or so ago.

Another Day in Rose's Life

The following week I received a telephone call from Rose asking the following question:

"Two mornings in a row I've been searching for two separate items that, in the end, I thought I'd lost. Both items appeared when I stopped looking. Yesterday I thought it was me - today I know it's not. I keep closing down, but I'm starting to feel drained and yesterday my flower was wilting. I am positive and have not let this bother me, but I need advice on how to strengthen this issue. I'm sorry - I feel like I'm bombarding you with so many questions."

"First of all," I said, "if you need to know the answer, then you must ask the question. Any form of doubt is a way to get to you, so you must feel sure in yourself as much as possible. The issue about things going missing is to create doubt in your mind. They can and will move and hide things to make you doubt yourself, so it's good to see that in the end you remained positive. It's not uncommon for things to turn up when you stop looking - it's like a game to them. When you stop looking, then they lose interest, because you're not getting frustrated that you can't find whatever it is that's missing. If you have a quick look and can't find something, let it go. If it's important, it'll turn up. That way you're not playing their game, so there'll be no point in them doing it any more. As far as closing down's concerned, you'll need to just run through what you're doing so I can check you're doing it right."

"I close my eyes and visualise my flower closing. Sometimes I have problems with the visualisation, so I start again. When I think I've got it right I then go on to visualising and expanding the white light to encompass all of me, then I ask my guides to help and protect me."

"So when you have trouble visualising your flower, what happens?"

"I get a sort of cobwebby cocoon surrounding me and I can't seem to focus on the flower."

"First you must take some deep breaths and be at peace with yourself. Concentrate on your breathing for a couple of minutes until you feel relaxed. When you've done that, then try to visualise your flower. If you still have trouble, then imagine the flower and try to imagine it closing. Believe in what you're doing, and remember your intention is to close down - keep that strong in your mind. Once you've closed your flower, then straight away imagine or visualise - whichever is easier - the white light at your feet and expand it to encompass your whole body. Once you're surrounded in the light, then ask your guides to help you to maintain your protection. There will be times to begin with when you'll have to go through the process a couple of times, but gradually it will get easier. When you've finished, trust in your guides to help you, and believe that you're protected. I know after a while you may feel the need to do it again - that's when subconsciously you're aware your protection has been breached. Don't concern yourself thinking you're not doing it properly. With the best will in the world, you have to remember that they will chip away until they find a weakness, so they can get at you again. You will gain strength with practice - you must now be aware of things more quickly and you'll know when things aren't right. This is you becoming more aware of the differences and recognising when you need to place protection around yourself again. That's how you're becoming stronger at the moment. Once you've conquered that, you'll find you've moved forward quite considerably."

"I'll try to do as you say. Thank you for listening to me and helping me."

"That's alright. Now get a good night's sleep and I'll see you at the church tomorrow night."

"Yes and thanks again. Bye."

The next day I called to check that everything was alright and Rose said:

"It's all just me - I'm feeling ill. I think I've got a virus. I'm sorry to give you all this hassle. I irritate myself at times. I apologise if I'm not at church tonight - it's because I'm ill and don't want to pass on this virus to anyone else."

"Tell me, when did you start feeling unwell and did it come on suddenly?"

"It was about lunch time. I suddenly felt my stomach was bloated and I was feeling sick. It must have been something I ate."

"This is another type of attack. If you suddenly feel unwell or have sudden pains, it's usually them giving you memories of past conditions. Once you recognise that, you'll find if you tell yourself it isn't yours, it will go away. It often happens to the sitters in my rescue circle - on the afternoon of the day we're going to sit, they sometimes get nasty headaches or stomach-aches. If they decide they're too ill to come and sit, when the time comes for the circle to start, they suddenly feel better and then they wish they'd come. It's the nasty spirits' way of stopping them from working. If, on the other hand, they come to the circle, then after we start they feel okay. What's happening is they don't want you near me, because they know I'll sense what's going on, and the more they can keep us apart, the easier they think it will be to beat you. Don't give in to it - come to the circle tonight and see for yourself. Even if you still feel ill, at least you'll know whether I'm right or not. I don't want you to work, but the energy that's produced in the circle will give your batteries a boost."

"Are you sure?"

"Yes. If you come along, you'll find out for yourself and if I'm wrong, you've lost nothing. When you see I'm right it'll give you a better idea of what you're up against, and what they're able to do."

"Alright, I'll see you later then."

That night when I arrived at the church, Rose was looking a bit down, so I asked her:

"How are you feeling?"

"I feel much better. My stomach doesn't hurt anymore, but I'm feeling a bit depressed because I'm not able to recognise what they're doing to me."

"Why would you expect to recognise something that you've always believed was you? After all, you weren't to know what they're capable of doing, were you? You should be proud of yourself - you've just beaten them again. As you said the other day, 'small steps': you can't expect to know all that's going on and how to deal with it. That's what I'm here for. Now come in and sit down. I don't want you to open up just sit and recharge your energies."

"I'll see how it goes."

During the circle everyone worked as normal and halfway through I asked everyone to join hands.

"Now I'd like you to feel the energy in the circle rotating from right to left, so as it comes from the person on your left, you'll pass it to the person on your right. You'll feel it getting stronger as it rotates. Draw it from the light in the middle of the circle and just let it build." After a couple of minutes I asked the sitters: "Now, starting with the person on Rose's right, let go of your hands."

One by one everyone let go, so that the energy passed through each of them and finally stopped at Rose. The sitters were quite surprised at how much they felt and Rose looked a lot better; in fact she was smiling.

"How do you feel now?" I asked her.

"That was wonderful. I would never have believed it was possible to get so much energy in that way."

"We'll do it again at the end of the circle just to strengthen it for you."

The circle only knew that Rose was feeling down; they didn't know the real reason behind what they had done. Some things must remain private to the individual. At the end, before we closed the circle, we did it again. Rose said she was feeling much stronger and more able to deal with whatever came next. I took Rose to one side and spoke quietly to her:

"Now remember, you're to think positive and trust in your guides to help you. If you need any extra help or explanation, then call me - I'm at the end of the phone. It doesn't matter what time it is - just phone. You'll still get things thrown at you and if you have any difficulty, then call me."

"I don't want to disturb you during the night. I'm sure it can wait until morning if anything happens."

"No, it's important that you call me at the time so we can deal with it then, otherwise you'll have more trouble with whatever it is the next time. Rest assured, it's not over yet. It's going to take a while and we must be ready to sort it out at the time."

"Alright, if you're sure. I just don't want to be a bother."

"You're no bother - it's what I do. If we're to beat them then we need to stay one step ahead all the time, so promise me you'll call if you need help."

"Okay, but I'll try not to. See you later."

"Bye for now."

Rose left and I went back to have a cup of tea and answer any questions that had come up in the circle. I then said my goodnights and left. I was feeling quite pleased with what had happened and was reassured that Rose was learning how to deal with things. She had been given the proof of what the nasty spirits were capable of, just by coming to the circle, and finding that the pains she had been getting were in fact memories, not real. The boost in energy that she had received would help her for a few hours at least, so I felt she would get through the night without too much trouble. She'd said she wasn't sleeping very well and one of the things we had to do was to regularise her sleep pattern so she would be more alert and able, should she need to be.

Rose's House

It was a week later that Rose telephoned to say she was having problems and she was quite upset. She was hearing noises, and getting feelings and sudden pains. She also felt there was someone watching her and was having trouble sleeping. I talked to her and decided it would be best if I went to see her and asked if that would be alright. She said:

"I didn't want to trouble you."

Again this sounds just like paranoid schizophrenia. It's such a shame there aren't more people who are able to tune in and support people who are going through this sort of thing.

"It's not a problem. I'll be there in half an hour. Is it alright if I bring my dog - you will find her reactions interesting."

"Yes that's fine," Rose replied.

When I arrived Rose was looking very tired and frightened. As I walked in, I immediately came under attack by nasty spirits and closed myself down so they couldn't get to me.

"So what's been happening?" I asked.

"I came home from work feeling a little tired but OK and when I walked in I suddenly felt drained and developed a splitting headache."

"Have you still got the headache?"

"Yes, I've taken some headache pills but they don't seem to be working."

"I can tell you the headache isn't yours. If I can just place my hand on your forehead it'll go very shortly."

I placed my hand on Rose's forehead and felt the energy around her: it was not nice. After about thirty seconds Rose's face brightened and she said.

"It's almost gone - what did you do?"

"I asked my guides to help me to remove the pain. You see you have nasty spirits around you, and one of the ways they get to you is to give you pain. As I've explained before, they can't give you what you've never had, but they can bring back the memories of pains you've had in the past. Sometimes all they have to do is come close enough so that you can feel their pain, if they have any. For example if you've never broken a leg you won't know what it feels like, so there's no memory for them to manipulate to cause you discomfort. However there are times, when they are very close to you, that you can pick up their ailments and think they are yours. This is how they work, by playing with your senses and feelings until they get you to a state where you don't know whether you're coming or going. Then they start playing with your mind while you're feeling low, so in the end you don't know what's yours and what isn't."

"So that's why I feel so drained?"

"Yes, they've attacked you as you walked in, before you could prepare yourself. So now we need to work through the things they've thrown at you and sort them out."

"I thought I was going mad. Is it really spirit or am I a nutcase?"

"Well, as to whether you're a nutcase, at this stage I've seen no evidence to support that. What I am aware of is that the spirits that are around you are intent on getting me away from you so they can continue to play. I'm being attacked at the moment but they're not getting through. What they're doing is trying to frighten me away so you will have no-one to turn to. It's not going to happen."

"Why do they do it? They must be really nasty to give people so much pain and discomfort."

"They do it partly because they can and partly because, if they don't, then they'll get it done to them. There are those in the spirit realms who are stronger than them and who're in control. As I said before, there are those who want power and the best way for them to get it is to show they're in control of not only those under their thumb, but also by showing others how they can control sensitive people like yourself. What are you feeling now?"

"I'm feeling very angry towards you. I don't want you here and I think you should leave. You're not welcome, you've misled me and I think you're trying to control me."

"That's interesting - they're making you feel antagonistic towards me to try to get you on your own so I can't help you. I will leave if you want me to. Because you've had this going on for a long time, you think this is normal. Which it is to you, but once we get rid of it you'll then realise the difference and you'll have your life back. At the moment you're being controlled by the nasty spirits that are here and who follow you around."

"You said you had got rid of them when you came to clear the house and when you came back to clear me, you said they had all gone."

"Yes and they had, but I also said you would need to protect yourself by closing down and not thinking of them, or what has happened. That would be like asking if they were still there - that is an invitation for others to come in and carry on where the others left off. Because you've had so much interference you don't know what normal is anymore, so you're not aware of them when they're around you, until they attack, by which time it's too late. Shall we start by getting you to close down and then we can get things under control again?"

"I still feel really angry with you and I think it would be better if you go."

"I will, but think about what I've just said and bear in mind, I'm aware of the spirits that are here and you're not making it up and or going mad. You've just gone very cold, haven't you?"

"Yes - how do you know?"

"Because I can sense what they're doing, now you're getting a little hyper and all of a sudden you're not tired and are feeling good about yourself?"

"Yes, that's what's happening."

"Yes, what they're doing is feeling confident now that I'm leaving, because they'll have you to themselves again. They really don't want me anywhere near you, as they know I'll help you to overcome them and get rid of them. But I will leave now if you're sure that's what you want."

"I don't know any more. Can you really get rid of them and are you sure I'm not going mad?"

"Yes, we can get rid of them and we have. Do you remember the first night, after we had finished, you had a peaceful night? That should show you it's not all in your mind. We can beat them, but it's your choice. Before you answer I'll warn you - because you're so sensitive it's not going to be an easy ride and you're going to have to fight. I will be there for you and help you, but at the end of the day it has to come from you. You have to exercise your free will and show them they're not wanted and block them out. It's up to you."

"If you are sure we can get rid of them I'll give it a try."

"No you have to mean it. We're not going to give it a try - we're going to succeed. One of the things they're going to do to you is make you feel insecure and undermine your feelings of self- confidence. They're also going to give you all sorts of feelings towards me and try to knock you off-balance. As I've said, they will not give up easily - they've had you in their pocket for too long to let go without a fight. I want you to be certain this is what you want, otherwise I'll leave and you can go back to how you were before all this started. You'll need courage, and you need to be able to trust in me. That will come as we progress and you see the changes in things around you. It's your decision. I will be quiet now while you think about it, or I can leave and give you more time to think."

"No, stay while I work things out. There are questions I need the answers to. If I decide to do this, you won't leave me high and dry, will you?"

"No, I am here for the duration, however long it takes."

"How long will it take?"

"Considering the strength of them, I would say they've been manipulating you for a long time, so it won't go away overnight. It's taken some time to get to this, so it will take a while to get rid of them. It also depends on how well you're able to close down and protect yourself. Don't expect it to all go away overnight - it's taken over a year before."

"Right - let's get started. What do we do first?"

"The first thing is to get you closed down and protected. I can lead you through but I can't do it for you because I would be interfering with your free will."

"What do I do?"

"First close your eyes - you may feel a little dizzy or feel a little sick. That's not you - that's just a way they have of trying to make you lose focus on what you're doing. Now concentrate on your breathing, breathe deeply and slowly at a pace that suits you. As you breathe, imagine you're very peaceful and in harmony with your body. Now we'll use a flower to close you down. You know in the evening the petals close up - picture that happening to your flower. As you do, believe in your heart that you're closed."

"I am trying, but I can't picture the flower."

"Right, just relax and concentrate on your breathing. Now we'll try a different meditation, as you're having trouble with this one. Imagine you're walking down a country lane; picture the hedges on either side; take notice of the leaves. Is there a slight breeze? Now smell the grass in the fields and listen; can you hear the sound of birds or other animals? Look at the sky - are there white clouds or is it overcast? Focus on these things and build up a reality in your mind of what you see, hear and smell. Have you been able to follow me?"

"I am getting a little dizzy and I am getting all sorts of feelings being thrown at me."

"Listen to what I say and concentrate on my voice. Picture the country lane and tell me what you see."

"I'm remembering a country lane I used to cycle down."

"That's good - now are you walking or cycling?"

"I'm cycling."

"Can you see the hedges on either side?"

"There's a hedge on one side and the other is open fields."

"That's good. Now can you see what's growing in the open fields?"

"They're just grass."

"Can you smell the grass?"

"I can smell something like wet grass."

"Good. Now look at the sky - what can you see?"

"It's a bit cloudy. It's been raining."

"Can you hear any birds or animals?"

"I can see some cows but I can't hear them."

"That's alright - what else is in your mind?"

"Nothing, just what I've told you."

"So you don't feel dizzy and you're not aware of anything else?"

"No, nothing."

"Open your eyes. That's a visualisation meditation: while your focus is on what you see or hear, your mind is under your control to the exclusion of everything else. Spirit will try to get in, but if you focus on what you're doing, they can't, and so can't give you their thoughts or interfere with yours. Each time you're aware of interference, try that meditation. Make it as real as you can. Be there."

"I had trouble at first, but once I focused on your voice it was easier and I was able to see the country lane. Once I saw that, the rest was easier."

"Good. Now in future when you feel uncomfortable, you must go through that routine from the breathing, to creating the pictures, to being there. Always believe you're in that place and nothing can interfere. It's no good just thinking it - you have to believe."

"I'll try, but it's not so easy without you talking me through."

"It will get easier as you become more proficient. Now we need to sort out this lot. Are you feeling better now?"

"Yes, I don't feel so angry or hyper now."

"Just accept the closing down has been done, and any time you feel or see something, ignore it. If you take no notice, they don't know whether they're getting to you or not until you react. So just ignore what they throw at you and if you can hang on, it'll go away. If you still have trouble, use your mind to focus on your visualisation. While you've got control of your mind it'll make it harder for others to get in."

"Do you mean the only way they know they're getting to me is by my reactions?"

"Yes, they can't feel what you're feeling because they're busy trying to mess with your feelings or emotions. If you don't react, they can't tell whether you're too strong or they're too weak to get through."

"So its mind games then?"

"Yes, because it's your mind they're playing with, not your body."

"Now I'm beginning to understand how they get through to me, maybe I can block them."

"Of course you can. It's just a matter of understanding what they're doing and counteracting it."

"What about the spirits in the house - aren't you going to remove them?"

"No. If you've done your protection properly, and you really understand how they're getting to you, they won't be able to bother you."

"Well I'm still frightened. I haven't slept very much for ages - what if they come back? Can you stay for a while so I have some feeling of security in case something happens?"

"Of course I will. You go to bed and try and sleep, and have a bit more confidence in your ability to block the thoughts. Focus on that meditation as you go to sleep. I'll be here if you need me and then if you get a problem I can deal with it. Is that alright?"

"That would make me feel a lot better. I'm sorry to make a fuss, but I am very frightened."

"That's okay. I told you I would help you and that's what I'm going to do. We can beat this."

It was one thirty and I sat on the sofa after wishing Rose good night thinking about how awful it must be to be so frightened to be alone. I was aware of the spirits around me and they weren't happy so I blocked them out and relaxed on the sofa. After about an hour Rose came out of her bedroom.

"I can't sleep I'm too frightened, every time I close my eyes I see horrible faces and I can't stop them."

"Come and sit here on the sofa and we'll see if we can't get rid of them for you."

I realised that because Rose had been getting these visions on a regular basis it was going to be difficult for her to fight them off initially. You see, if you expect them, they will come, and as Rose had been getting them most nights, she would need support in overcoming them. She sat on the end of the sofa and I placed my hands on her shoulders to give her healing to calm her down. While I was doing this I got the thought from my guides that we should help her to sleep. By giving her healing until she was so relaxed she fell asleep. This is what they did and after ten minutes she seemed to be asleep, as much from exhaustion as from healing. I covered her up and went and sat in the armchair where I could keep an eye on her. She slept for about 6 hours and woke with a start, she saw me and was immediately apologetic.

"I'm so sorry I fell asleep when you were giving me healing you can't be very comfortable there."

"It's of no concern the armchair's very comfortable, how did you sleep?"

"I just went out like a light and didn't know anything until I woke just now."

"Good are you feeling a little better now?"

"Yes. I'm still tired but not as frightened as I was last night. I'm sorry you've been here all night - aren't you tired?"

"A little weary, but it's not the first time I've stayed up, and I'm sure it won't be the last. Now why don't you sort yourself out and then I suggest a nice walk, to get away from this atmosphere and clear your head - it'll make you feel better."

How it Began

Rose went and had a bath and got dressed, then she insisted on cooking some breakfast. After eating, we went for a walk along the beach for a couple of hours. While we walked I asked her about her beliefs, and what she understood about the spirit world.

"Well I've been thinking this all started when I was about ten years old," she said. "We used to live in a flat which was always cold. I used to get the feeling I was being watched all the time, and sometimes when I looked in the mirror I saw horrible eyes looking at me. I thought I was seeing things, but after a while I realised - even then - that I only saw the eyes at home. If I went to a friend's, I felt warm and relaxed. When I went home I sort of tensed up and started feeling that I didn't want to be there. Over the years things have changed, but the basics are still the same. Is it because my mum played with the Ouija board, or is it because I did? Is that why I'm getting all this?"

"It's both, "I said. "When you play with the Ouija board you can get spirits attaching themselves to you by invading your aura. Once they're there, it's very hard to shift them. Some of them don't know that you are feeling their discomfort - they are just looking for help. There are others who know what they are doing and will then work on controlling you or just messing with your emotions. Plus the fact that you're very sensitive to energies around you, and that's why we have to get you closed down."

"Thinking back, I remember that I've had these voices chattering in my head for years and I can't stop them. I have a man who is pure evil and menacing who's playing strong mind games. It's in my mind all the time and I can't stop looking in the mirror. It's as though I'm drawn to the mirror, and I just stare into it. I have an evil smirk on my face at times and I can't stop it. I had a lot of children this morning and when I say go away, the chatter gets worse. I can't remember not having this chatter. I'm doing my best to stay positive and strong with the understanding this is an illusion, but I'm unable to block the presence that's behind me. I know I'm not mad, but what with one thing and another it's hard to stay strong sometimes. Over the years I've had an interest in many things, and some of them I feel have helped me to understand more about myself."

"It's not an illusion: spirit is real. The chatter you hear is from spirit, and while most people can't or don't tune in to that frequency, there are many that do. Those that admit to hearing voices are often diagnosed as schizophrenic and put on drugs to dull the mind so that the voices go away. Those drugs can and do cause problems to the brain as the doses get stronger. As the body gets used to the drugs, the doctors just change them or give stronger doses. It's not a cure, as they won't accept that there is more to this life than most people can see or believe. There are a lot of people who are in mental institutions exhibiting the same problems you're getting."

"I feel for them - drugs don't solve anything. I know. I've been there in a different way."

"Tell me what's taken your interest."

"Well, I got very involved in crystal healing and the power of crystals. I have quite a collection and I know most of the properties of each crystal, you know, when to use them and what for. I trained to Reiki 2 with healing and self- healing with a Reiki master, and I have learnt from meditation tapes how to raise my vibrations to the highest level. I've also taken a course in aromatherapy, and reflexology and have my diplomas. I found that, as I learnt, I was able to find my peace and was able to put things in perspective. I also get a lot of comfort from my angel cards and meditations."

"Why did you stop your meditations?"

"I just didn't have the time, or I wasn't feeling very well and I would have trouble focusing."

"So, like all meditations, if you aren't focusing to the exclusion of everything else, they can be interfered with. You should continue with the meditations that work for you. Everyone is different - if it works, use it."

"I found I could get to a very high vibration by doing meditations with my crystals and angel cards. You don't believe in angels, do you?"

"When you say 'angel', do you mean with wings?"

"No, just a spirit I suppose, from the higher realms. Do you believe in angels?"

"To me, there are guides who look after me and my spirit, and then what I call overseers. They look on from a distance and coordinate my spiritual pathway with others, who think or work in the same way that I do. You see, my guides look after my immediate situation, and the overseers have a much wider view of where I'm going, and they help me to make the right spiritual connections with others on the earth plane. If you like, they see a much bigger picture of my journey, and help my guides in planning the next step. At the end of the day it doesn't make any difference as long as it works for you - it's just a different name for the same thing. It's interesting that you're interested in healing. I wonder if, maybe at some stage, you opened up and never closed properly after giving healing. It's quite possible you picked up something that has attached itself to you. There are a lot of persistent nasty spirits around you. Because you're particularly sensitive, they're getting through to you any time they want. That's why you have to learn to close down and stay closed."

"When I was feeling good about myself and able to tune in to the higher realms, I felt drawn to go to the local spiritualist church. I would go and have healing and found I could pick up on spirit, and I was able to give messages to the healers. The healing leader said I shouldn't do that - if I wanted to develop, then I should attend the open circle. I've always had an interest since as long as I can remember, but it wasn't until about four years ago I first sat in an open circle. During the meditation, I saw a man with a flat cap. He just flashed into my awareness and sat there smiling. I remembered I had seen him before on a number of occasions. I was told by the circle leader that he was my doorkeeper. He seems to follow me around. I've seen him at work too, but then I see him like I see you. What do you think about him?"

"Well, in the first place he's a short tubby man from about 1930s England, isn't he, and when he comes in he comes from the front and just appears. Is that right?"

"Yes, that's how I see him."

"First of all, you must remember we choose our guides from friends we know when we're in spirit. They're spirits we've been working with, or know of, when we decide it's time to take another journey through life. As this man could only have died in the last 60 or 70 years, he can't possibly be a guide."

"Why not? He seems to know what he is doing."

"Yes, but do you? When we pass to spirit it will take a couple of hundred years before we would even think about returning. That's because we'll want to make sure our loved ones are safely back home to the spirit world before we move on. If you take into account our children and grandchildren, then it's going to be a while before they're all safely back. On top of all that, we still have to adjust to our true selves and the knowledge of who and what we are. You're not 'Rose' in the spirit world - that's just the label that's been put on you in this life. You're far more than that. The nasty spirits don't go through that process because they don't go back to heaven - they stay in the spirit realms around the earth. There are many reasons why they don't go to heaven. They may get lost and then waylaid by others who are already in the spirit realms. You see nasty spirits are just as abundant in the spirit realms as they are here. Just because they've passed over doesn't mean they've changed: they have to want to, just like here. If they get caught by other nasty spirits they'll be restricted and taught how to do things to people here, and then made to do it. Imagine being lost and someone finding you and offering to help you - you would be grateful if they took you under their wing and looked after you, wouldn't you?"

"Yes, but if they're nasty, why don't our guides find us first or stop them from capturing us?"

"Our guides are there with us, but usually we either don't see them or don't recognise them as such. It can be pretty confusing to find there is something else, when all your life you believed that when you died there was nothing. It's just as bad for people who have been devout in their faith and believe or expect someone like God or Jesus to be waiting for them. They're also going to be confused when they find there's no-one like that there. Sometimes they think they've sinned and are being left in the spirit realms, where it's cold and dark, to atone for their sins before they can be collected and taken on.

As I said before, we're still going to use our eyes to see when we get over there, unless we've been acclimatised by our loved ones, who gather round when we're on our deathbeds. If someone has more of an understanding, such as you and I, of what to expect, then there is little likelihood that we will have that kind of problem. Until people learn about life after death, and realise you see with your senses, there will always be people that get lost. Your guides are not allowed to stop the nasty spirits from capturing you, or force themselves on you, because of free will. It's like most things here - if you don't ask, how does anyone know what you need?

There are those who feel they've had a rough ride through life and want revenge, or are angry with someone on the earth plane and want to find a way to get back at them. What they don't realise is that when they get to the spirit realms, a thought is all it needs to move them from one place to another. If you find yourself in a strange place that's not nice, your thought may be to get away from there, but as you don't know where to go, you will arrive somewhere just as unsettling. Then there are the nasty spirits who will move you to a place of their choosing so they can manipulate you. If you don't know where you are and don't know where you have come from, it's very difficult, if not impossible, to find your way to anywhere, as you don't have a point of reference to work from. So if your plan was to get back at maybe someone in your family or an acquaintance, you'll find it very difficult because how are you going to find them? Many people think that if someone died in a house they will haunt it - that's very unusual because, until they get to heaven and regain their spirit memories, they will not be able to find their house or family. That's why the nasty spirits have so much control over those who are lost. They really are lost: if they only knew they could ask their guides for help at any time, then they would be taken to heaven and wouldn't have to suffer or wait to be rescued."

"Why can't people, when they die, just go to heaven?"

"Most do - it's only a very few that don't. You have to remember there's no time in spirit, so if someone gets lost they can be lost for hundreds of years. Because it's always now and they're not aware of the passing of time, there's no urgency with them to try and sort things out."

"So he can't be a guide, then, from what you've said?"

"No, your guides are from a lot further back than that. It takes quite a few of our years to learn the skills that are needed to look after the soul of another while they're on their journey through life. They may have learnt their skills hundreds of years ago and been back for another life after that. They won't come as a guide to anyone until they've sorted out the lessons they received while on the earth."

"So if we see someone who isn't from at least two hundred years ago, they can't possibly be a guide, even though they may have learnt how to be one before their last life?"

"That's right, because they want to see their loved ones safely home first."

"So what's a doorkeeper, then?"

"There are two ways of looking at guides - one is that you have a doorkeeper who monitors who comes forward, depending on what you're doing. This doorkeeper is with you all the time and only lets your other guides come in when you need them. Then there's the other way of looking at it, which is that your guides will come forward to work with you when you need their expertise. They rotate their duties so there is always someone there, but when you're developing and you get to know some of your guides, they'll always be there while you're working. That way, you can build a bond with them and learn to get to know them and trust them. Neither way is wrong - it just depends on what you're comfortable with. But for me, I let my guides choose who is most suitable for the work I'm doing."

"I've always believed in a doorkeeper. It makes me feel more comfortable, knowing someone is looking after me."

"That's all very well if the spirit you see as a doorkeeper is indeed a guide. If they're not, then they won't let any of your guides come through."

"Can't my other guides just come in when I need them?"

"Not if you've accepted the wrong spirit as a doorkeeper, because he will only invite his friends in. Because of free will, your guides can't do anything about it until you do."

"So how do I know if my doorkeeper is right?"

"You won't, unless you find a medium who can sense when they're right or wrong."

"But you can do that, can't you?"

"Yes, but I would never interfere with your beliefs. Unless somebody asks, I would never tell them whether their guide or doorkeeper was right or wrong. I work by the same rules my guides do: if you want to know, you must ask. If you ask, then there must be some doubt as to whether who you've got is right."

"So the man with the flat cap isn't my doorkeeper then, is he?"

"No, he's not. As I explained, he can't be a guide because he's not from far enough back. Tell me what happened in the open circle."

"When we were asked to give each other a reading, I got some good results. That encouraged me to continue going. I thought I had found the place where I could develop. I was doing quite well except for one person who was quite good at readings, I could never get anything right with him. It was only him, no-one else. When I think back, even when I was a little child I always knew who to stay away from - I would pick up their negativity. That's one of the reasons I try to stay away from crowded places like shops and markets. I just seem to draw people's negative feelings. Anyway, I was going to the open circle and gradually things started to go wrong. I went to an evening of transfiguration at a lady's house. While I was sitting, I got something that made me feel awful. Next thing I know, they're all standing around me, giving me healing. I felt terrible after that night and stopped going to the church. Things seemed to get worse and for about two years after that I had loads of problems and nothing seemed to go right."

"From what you've said, it seems fairly obvious that you had a spirit attach itself to you. If the people who were there had known what they were doing, they would have realised what had happened and cleared it. A lot of people get problems from going to, or running, evenings or groups for things they know little about. There are a lot of mediums who don't believe in negative spirits: from what you say, their answer was to give you healing."

"That's when I got involved with crystals and they seemed to make me feel better. But I was still getting major changes in my emotions for no apparent reason. It would take days for me to balance myself again. No sooner had I got myself on an even keel, it would start all over again."

"Did these changes come over you suddenly?"

"Sometimes I would realise things had changed around me and then realise what was happening, and sometimes it would happen all of a sudden."

"I see. So what you're saying is you were getting the same sort of thing, but sometimes you were aware of it straight away and sometimes it would take a while before you realised?"

"Yes, but in either case I was not able to control my feelings. That's why I've had trouble with relationships both with partners and family. I just find fault for no reason and what was a good relationship starts to fall apart. I don't get on with my sister and have always had trouble with my mum. She's always putting me down and has never encouraged me in anything. When I try to help her with things, she just says 'here we go, Rose knows best', and all I'm doing is trying to help."

"So generally your life is pretty isolated?"

"Yes, and every time I try to change it, things start going wrong again. It's as if someone is trying to stop me from enjoying life. After a few years I had got myself in a better state of mind and went back to the spiritualist church and sat in the open circle again. I also went to a few workshops and was starting to enjoy myself again, then I was asked if I would like to join a closed circle. I said yes and for a couple of weeks things seemed to be going fine then on the third week it all fell apart again - as you know, because you were running the circle."

"Yes and you've been having the same sort of problems that you experienced last time you came to the church. The only difference is that I'm helping you now and I'm able to detect what is - and what is not - spirit."

"Do you really think you can sort this out?"

"I know we can sort this out. Together we'll work our way through the different type of attacks and deal with them one at a time. As you gain more of an understanding of what's happening, it'll be easier for you to recognise things and so block them. It's a case of going slowly and understanding what the nasty spirits are doing and how it's affecting you, then helping you to deal with it."

"I have to tell you there was a time that I couldn't handle the voices and took to drugs to try and block them out."

"Did it work?"

"For a time, then it all came back again. In the end I decided that wasn't the route to go down and stopped. It took a while and I had to see the doctor, who sent me to see a psychiatrist."

"What did they have to say?"

"They said there was a chance that I had schizophrenia and they wanted to put me on tranquillizers. I took them for a while, but they just made me feel dozy and I just couldn't get on with anything."

"What did you do?"

"I weaned myself off and once my head was clear I took an interest in angel cards and crystals again. They helped me immensely with meditations and by attuning myself with the crystals I felt much better. You don't believe in that sort of thing, do you?"

"It's not for me to question your beliefs. It doesn't matter what I believe - it's what works for you that counts. If you find these things give you comfort, then who am I to say they're wrong. Just as long as you believe in something. It's the belief that counts, that's what spirit is all about - everything they do is done with belief. They say that thoughts are living things, well in spirit it is the intent behind the thought that makes it work."

"Is that why things got better for me, because I believed in what I was doing?"

"Yes, however, it's plain to see there are areas that still have to be dealt with. You can't have nasty spirits bothering you all the time, so we have to deal with it."

"I do find it hard to stay closed. Sometimes I think I haven't closed down properly and sometimes I get a lot of interference when I'm trying to close down."

"I know it's not easy to start with and especially after they have more or less done what they want. As I said, they won't give up easily- we'll have to fight to get rid of them. When you say you get interference, what do you get exactly?"

"When I'm trying to close down, I try using the flower with its petals closed and next thing I know they're open again. Then if I manage that and go on to picture a white light, sometimes it just fades away and sometimes there's something blocking me from seeing it. It doesn't matter what I try, I can't picture it, so I have trouble when I try to expand it to surround me. If I can't see it, how do I know if I've done it properly?"

"It doesn't matter whether you see it or feel it - what matters is your intention. They may stop you from seeing the flower, but if you truly believe it, then it will happen. What you have to understand is that thoughts and beliefs are real things in the spirit realms, just the same as if you paint a picture here: it's real. The difference is that, in the spirit realms, you create things by thought, not with your hands. Once you can get to that stage, then your white light is no different. Believe it and it will happen."

"I also get words in my mind. I don't know what they are, but it's like a lot of chatter and I can't stop it."

"I've shown you a guided meditation where you are going through fields and seeing, feeling and smelling what's around you. If you can sit down and do that when you hear the chatter, or even follow one of your angel meditations, it will help you regain control of your mind and the chatter will stop. You may have to do it a number of times, but remember each time you do, you're saying to all who are taking notice of you that you don't want to work with the nasty spirits - only your guides."

"What if I get a sudden attack? I won't have a chance to close down."

"Let's deal with each situation as it happens, then you'll know how to handle it if it occurs again."

"I'm beginning to understand, but there's so much to learn. I wonder if I will ever be able to get this under control."

"Of course you will. As I've said, there will be ups and downs, but you will see your progress by looking back at how things used to be. Now, are you going to be alright or do you want me to stay and keep an eye on you?"

"I think I'll be okay now."

I knew she was going to be alright for the rest of the day, as Rose told me she was going to a friend's wedding reception, and staying with another friend for the night.

"Just try not to drink too much and stay in control of your emotions and you should be alright," I said.

Rose said she didn't drink much anyway and was quite positive she would be okay.

Picking up Negative Energies

I spoke to Rose on the telephone the next afternoon and asked her how she was doing. She said:

"When I go to the supermarket, I pick up negative feelings from other shoppers as I go round. When I've finished my shopping I feel drained, as if all the energy has been taken out of me. I feel tired and irritable and can't seem to shake it off. I go home and try to meditate to change my energy and give myself some positive energy, but it only works some of the time. If it doesn't work I get moody and then get depressed, and it can take me days to sort myself out again."

"What appears to be happening is you pick up on other people but you only pick up the negative," I said. "This suggests to me that you're being guided to the negative side of life by those in spirit who want to control you. Once they get you on a downward spiral, it's much easier for them to then hit you with other feelings like tiredness and irritability. I expect you also get pains either in your head like headaches, or pains in your stomach. These are quite easy to bring up from your memory as most people have had one or the other at some time. Women are more likely to get stomach pains than men, because of their biological make-up. When the spirits continually hit you with different things like that, they'll get you to a state where you just curl up and hope it goes away. It's very difficult to find your way out of that kind of situation on your own, which is why another person, who is able to tune in to what's going on, can help."

"I seem to pick up negative energies from people at work as well. In fact, everywhere I go where there are a number of people."

"That's because you are what is termed a highly sensitive person. It's not a disease - it's just the way you are. There are hundreds of people like you and some doctors are starting to recognise the symptoms. It can be difficult to overcome these feelings or block them and when you've got spirit annoying you as well it just makes it harder, as you will be trying to decide where it's coming from. Just treat it all as the same problem and protect yourself in the usual way. In some cases it may be easier, as you can sometimes see who it's coming from. When you know who is sending it out, you can put a barrier around yourself to deflect their emotions. They won't necessarily realise what they are doing: ninety-nine percent of the time it just happens when they are feeling a bit down."

"So, not only have I got spirits to deal with but people as well?"

"Yes, I'm afraid so. While you are learning to deal with the spiritual side you will automatically build up your ability to deal with the earthly negativity as well."

"I suppose if I'm aware of where it's coming from, at least I've got a chance of dealing with it."

Rose said she was feeling better about things now we had had a chat, so we said goodbye and hung up.

The Rescue Circle

Rose came round on the Sunday on her way home, just to let me know she was alright. When she walked in I offered her a cup of tea and she said there was a lot of energy around us.

"Yes," I said. "This is where I run my rescue circle."

"What do you do in your rescue circle?" Rose asked.

"I'm teaching some friends how to help lost souls and remove nasty spirits that out guides bring to our circle."

"How do you do that?"

"First I teach them how to communicate with their guides and introduce them to one guide to start with. Then I teach them to trance, that is a light trance where they're aware of what is going on and are in control of what happens. Then I teach them how to recognise who's coming through before they get there. That's done by asking their guides to come through, and monitoring their guides, until they're through and they start to speak. I will often let them get the wrong spirit through and then question them afterwards, to see if they realise whether it was right or not. It's quite easy to tell the difference, as the guide will have their own way of speaking. When you know someone well, you recognise them from how they speak or the phraseology they use. It's no different with guides and imposters, except you can also sense when it isn't right. You see, their guides will always come through gently and slowly - they will never just appear. If, while the guide is coming forward, a nasty spirit jumps in, then the guide will allow it, to teach the medium the lesson of recognition and control. Our guides work on a strict law of free will: if the medium lets someone else other than their guide in, they have to show the rest of the nasty spirits who're watching that they don't want them there by throwing them out. It will happen in all sorts of ways, until the medium learns to focus on their guide, and not allow anyone else to come through. In that way they also learn to bring the nasty spirits through, and control them, until we have spoken to them, and dealt with them accordingly."

"Why do you need to bring the nasty spirits through?"

"Its good practice, so that when we go to someone's house like we did yours, we're able to sort out who is nasty and remove them. We can then help the lost souls to get back home to their loved ones safely. We've now been sitting for about a year and we're quite busy on circle nights, sorting out those who are lost and helping them, and getting rid of the nasty spirits who try to disrupt our circle."

"Is that why I felt so much energy here when I came in?"

"Yes. What happens is that our guides are busy all week finding lost souls and bringing them here for us to help when we sit. It's good practice for us and we're helping our guides to rescue those who are lost. Because of the work we do, a big beacon of light has appeared above this house so other lost souls can find us as well. It's like a spotlight in the dark and all who see it are either curious, or want to interfere with what's going on."

"So it's not just lost spirits that come here, then?"

"No, the problem with having such a big light is it attracts both good and bad, the former for help and the latter because they think it will be easy pickings for them, to capture the lost souls. If the bad guys can disrupt us, then we'll spend more time getting rid of them and less time helping the others. We try to get rid of the nasty spirits fairly quickly, so we can get on with the real work, which is rescue. We have to talk to the nasty spirits briefly to find out if they want to go to heaven - if they do, then we take them."

"Why can't your guides rescue the lost souls? After all, they bring them here so why can't they take them straight to heaven and get rid of the nasty spirits?"

"Everyone, good or bad, is entitled to go to heaven. They must all be given a choice, that way they all have free will. If they don't want to go, then we just place them in a bubble of white light, where they stay because they can't get out. Our guides then talk to them and try to help them to understand what they are doing is wrong. We'll try to persuade them and even enclose them in a bubble of spiritual light in the hope that they'll see reason and go to the light. Sometimes they'll go and sometimes they won't. If they do want to go, then we protect them and take them to heaven. Our guides can rescue lost souls, but what takes about five minutes for us to do, can take spirit nine months. That's one of the reasons we use light trance, because when we bring the spirit through, they feel a difference. That is, they feel the weight of the body, which they haven't realised is gone until we bring them through. On top of that, we're able to talk to the lost souls, who are still focused on the earthly and so can see us, but can't see spirit. As I told you before, it's not until we tell them to open their eyes that they actually open their senses and become aware of the spirit world. Another reason for bringing them through is so that when we go to someone's house, they can hear what's being said. It helps with their understanding of what's been going on in their home. As for the nasty spirits, most of them know they only have to ask and they will be taken to heaven, but they have to ask - again, it's free will. Some of them have been to heaven and left because they were bored and it's more fun for them to mess around with people like yourself."

"What's a bubble? I've heard you talk about it, and when you were at my house, you put some nasty spirits a bubble. What does it do?"

"Well, as I said, we can't take away free will even from the nasty spirits, but we can make it more difficult for them to do what they do. A bubble is an energy field that we put around them and it does two things. It stops them from interfering with spirits and people on the earth plane. And because it's a calming energy, it helps them to relax. When they have had time to think, our guides will then talk to them and try to help them to see reason."

"If that's the case, how come the problems I was getting after you had thrown out the nasty spirits from my house continued?"

"What you have to remember is that you have an aura which can be read by spirit and some mediums. Everything that has happened to your soul is in that aura and can be read. It's easier for the nasty spirits to carry on with what they know works than to start over again, so they just copy what's been done before. That's what makes it difficult for people if they get the aggravation back again. They think it's the same ones who're doing it. That undermines our credibility and people don't believe we've cleared them, so they try to live with it and so the problem goes on."

"Why can't you just clear things and make sure the same problem can't come back?"

"We do, but it depends on how susceptible the individual is, and whether they listen to what we're telling them about how to close down and get on with their lives. If they're too open then it takes a while for them to get to grips with it. Take yourself, for instance. You're so sensitive - we can't take that away from you, so I have to teach you other ways to combat the problem. You're quite rare in that you're more sensitive than most, therefore your job is going to be harder to get it under control, and so will take longer. I've been to so many houses where they've been having problems and we've been able to resolve them. Most of them were people who had no connection or interest in spirit. They were just in the wrong place at the wrong time. But there have been others who've been involved who have had an interest: some we've managed to help and others, who know best, have still got their problems. I'm not saying we're always right - there's still so much to learn - but most of the latter are too headstrong, or are being told by another medium to do other things, and because they're listening to them, they're still troubled. There've been those who've had medical problems who, although we can remove the spirits, either don't want to be alone (any attention is better than none), or their mind is not quite right, so the problem continues, because they can't control it. Some of these people do need medication, but others are just lonely and crave company. We also have to consider the effects of the drugs they're taking as these can be mind-numbing, which means the person hasn't either got the willpower or the determination to fight. Those we're unable to help, but you're none of these - you're just ultra -sensitive, so we have to deal with your situation in a different way."

As I was talking, I felt a prickly feeling around my head, so I suggested to Rose that we take a short walk, the idea being to change the energy around her before the nasty spirits attacked her. When we left the house she seemed to perk up and we had a walk along the seafront for about half an hour.

Sensitivity

After we got back we talked about Rose's sensitivity. This was going to cause her some problems, and we had to look at other ways for her to get things under control.

"Because you're so sensitive to other people and energies, closing down is only part of your protection," I said. "We need to look at other ways that you can protect yourself."

"This is going to be difficult, isn't it?"

"No just a learning curve, if you like. A re-education to your particular understanding and sensitivity."

"What do you do to close down?"

"Well I close down by just turning off to spirit, if things are busy, then I place protection around myself. It stops most of it, but then I just ignore anything I become aware of and just get on with what I'm doing. It's what you believe, as much as what you do to protect yourself. To be fair, I have perfected my protection over a period of thirty years and I've had to change how I do things as I've progressed."

"So you had similar problems to me in the beginning?"

"Yes, but I wasn't as sensitive as you back then. It's only as I've learnt, that I've become more in tune with spirit. But I've also learnt to turn it all off if I want to, so that it doesn't bother me. I seem to be able to tune in when I'm working and tune out when I'm not. I can't really say how I do it - let's just say it works for me, so I don't question it."

"So you're saying the closing down is just part of the protection. I thought you said it would be all I needed to do."

"Under normal circumstances, yes, but it's your sensitivity that causes the problem. We have to take things one at a time and see how it affects you. We can then work out the best way for you to defend yourself. You're already starting to be aware of when things are changing. Now we just need to put up a defence before they get in to you."

"I'm not always aware of the nasty spirits until it's too late, and it's changed somehow. I was starting to notice a change and now I find it harder."

"That's because it's more subtle now, and as you get better at it, it will become even more subtle. But as you progress, so you'll become more sensitive to their games and stop them before they can get a hold on you. Yes, there will be times when you get it wrong, but don't think of it as a failure - more as a lesson. I could tell you how to stop a lot of things happening, but until it happens to you, there's no point as you won't remember everything. So we must deal with each attack as it comes."

"So the fact that I'm picking up on spirits in your house means I'm becoming more sensitive?"

"No you've always been this sensitive. It's because we're talking about it that you're aware of what's going on around you. Ordinarily you would be as closed as you're going to get, but your senses are heightened at the moment."

As if to prove the point Rose's face started to change and she looked as though she was frightened.

"Okay let's go into the kitchen and make a cup of tea," I said. I took Rose by the arm and guided her into the kitchen.

"Was I going off again?" she asked.

"They were getting close, so I thought a change of energy around you would help - that's why we've come into the kitchen."

"So it's as easy as that to stop them?"

"Sometimes. We just have to see what's going to work for you. Then when you're aware of a change, you can do something positive that requires your thoughts."

"Is it going to be like this for the rest of my life?"

"No, just until it becomes second nature and you find what works for you. Over a period of time you'll find you're blocking things automatically and you won't even give it a thought."

"Why is it so hard for me, when other people seem to be able to control it without any problem?"

"Other people don't have your history or sensitivity. There are a lot of people who are sensitive, who've been sectioned and put in psychiatric institutions by those who don't understand mediumship. You see, depending on who you're talking to, depends on whether its mediumship or schizophrenia. They hear voices and see things as well, but it's not always understood by those around them who don't."

"In that case most mediums should be locked up as well."

"That's the point. There are many mediums who are lucky enough to learn how to control what they're getting. It's those who can't - or haven't learnt - who have the problems."

We talked a while and Rose reminded me about the constant chatter she used to have in her head, and how the only way she could stop it was to get drunk. After a while, even that didn't stop it and she took to drugs. That worked for a while but she realised that wasn't the answer. When she was lucid the chatter came back and she decided to stop taking drugs. It took her a couple of years to clean herself up, but she hadn't taken any now for about five years or more. She still gets the chatter but not so often, and now that she's learning to close down, it's even less often. Because of her sensitivity, the nasty spirits have had a field day with her emotions, but we're now making it more difficult for them. While we were talking I was aware of an uncomfortable feeling around Rose, so I said to her, 'focus on what you're saying - there are some spirits around you'. Just as I finished saying that, her eyes changed, they became dull and vacant and she started to giggle. I knew there was a nasty spirit with her, so I left her for a moment to see if she could get it under control. When she couldn't, I started talking to her about how she was much stronger than them, and she needed to fight and not to give in. It was obvious she hadn't been aware of them coming close, because she hadn't been able to try and block them. Gradually her eyes cleared and she became upset.

"It happened again, didn't it? Is it because we were talking about them that they were able to get in? Was my mind open because I was thinking about them?"

"There is a strong possibility that when we talk about things that have happened to you, you're remembering the experience that you had, and that makes it easier for them to influence you. They've gone now and you managed to come back a lot quicker than last time, so you're getting better. Don't worry, I said it will take time and there's a lot of improvement since we first met."

"But I can't tell when they're there until afterwards and then it's too late."

"That's not true. If you think about it, you're much more aware of when they're attacking you with your emotions. It's only a matter of time before you get this under control as well."

Knowing how frightened Rose was about getting caught again and bearing in mind that when she was on her own, it had taken hours for her to come back sometimes, Rose was worried about going home in case she was attacked again. I told her she would be alright: even if she was attacked, she would learn something and be stronger next time. Rose went home having closed down and, having a positive mind, we were sure she would be able to cope. The reason she was getting attacked more frequently was simply because she was fighting to get rid of them and they didn't want to let go.

I knew we would have this problem: as Rose was so sensitive, it would take a while to get things in order. Rose telephoned me about lunchtime the next day as I had asked her to.

"How are you getting on today?" I asked.

"I have been up and down. There's a women who sits opposite me and she can be quite negative and I keep picking up her negativity. That makes me negative and I then start getting angry. I know it's not me, but I can't seem to shake it off."

"You need to build a wall in your mind between you and her. If she speaks to you and she's being negative, take a deep breath before you answer. That way, you won't say anything that might make her worse. You need to try and tune her out of your mind. If it gets too bad, then go for a walk or something to change your energy. Remember, take some deep breaths to calm yourself each time you feel a little agitated. You have to keep your emotions from going up or down as much as possible."

"I'll try. I'm out of the office at the moment doing a little errand. It gives me a chance to get away from all the negativity."

"Good. Another thing you can do is say something nice if she's uptight, and see how that affects her disposition - you'll be surprised at the difference it can make when someone is a little prickly. Most importantly, don't allow her to put her problems on you: because of your sensitivity you tend to take on board other people's problems. You can't do anything to help them, so let them sort it out for themselves. You would be surprised how many people unload their problems on others, and then walk away feeling better. They may not know what they're doing, but you can bet your boots a lot of them do. You're like a piece of blotting paper - you just absorb the negativity, and then it's no wonder you feel as if you've got everyone's problems on your shoulders. It's too much for one person. You have to let it slide off and get on with your own life. Sometimes you can care too much about others and it'll drag you down, that's one of the problems with being sensitive."

Rose said she would give it a try and rang off.

Later that Evening

That evening Rose called me about 11 o'clock to ask for some advice.

"When I got home, I was feeling quite good but as the evening has progressed, things have gone downhill," Rose said.

"What's been happening?" I asked.

"When I came in, the house felt a bit cold. I thought it was because I hadn't been here. After I had something to eat, I settled down to do some studying and I could feel myself getting more and more irritated. I thought about it, but there was nothing to annoy me, so I decided to ignore it, as I felt I was being attacked. I had already closed down before I came into the house so, taking your advice, I just moved to the sofa and carried on with my studying. After about half an hour I was starting to get very angry at you, I don't know why, but I hated you and never wanted to talk to you again. I even thought it was you that was making me angry. I stopped studying and went for a bath, and when I got in the bath I started hearing noises - you know, like there was someone in the house walking up and down. I knew there wasn't anybody there because the door was locked and I live on my own. I tried to convince myself it was just nasty spirits and they could do no harm, just make a noise. I just got out of the bath as calmly as I could and went into the bedroom and got ready for bed. When I got into bed I had the feeling that there was someone sitting on the other side of the bed watching me. So I turned over and closed my eyes. There were a lot of faces being put in my head and as soon as I got rid of them by thinking of something nice, I started seeing eyes. Not normal eyes but red ones, really close. I put on some music and tried to listen to that. The next thing I know it's half an hour later and I'm feeling awful. I think I've been taken away again and I don't know how to stop it. I did everything you told me to but I couldn't stop it. Am I mentally ill?"

"No - if you were you wouldn't be able to rationalise what's happened. Are you alright now?"

"I seem to have calmed down while I have been talking to you, but if this is going to keep happening, how am I going to lead a normal life?"

"It's not going to keep happening. If you think back, you didn't even know it had happened most of the time, so you're progressing. Gradually you'll be able to sense when things are getting heavy and be able to change your thoughts and stop it from happening. It's a slow process, but by sticking to your guns we will win. Just don't give up on yourself. I know you wonder sometimes whether you can beat them, but remember, you're now recognising what is, and isn't your thoughts. That's a big step in the right direction. Just keep at it and trust in what you think. Always rationalise a situation or a thought and you'll see most of the thoughts that aren't yours won't be logical. Always think it through and you'll see the truth. Now are you going to be okay? Is there anything else you want to talk about or tell me?"

"No I think I'm okay. I just needed to talk to you and get some understanding of what's going on. That's the first time anything has been thrown at me and it freaked me out a bit."

"Well you handled it very well. Try to remember to stay calm whatever is happening and trust that your guides are with you, and no physical harm will come to you. As I said before, it's all mind games - they're just playing with your head to try and get control of you. If you let them, they'll start to control your life again so don't give in, take control."

"So they're going to be in the house all the time. It's just a case of me learning to control my thoughts and not letting them take over again?"

"Yes, to a degree. Once they realise you're not such an easy target, they'll move on to someone that's not such hard work. They're lazy and will only work on people they can get to. Surely you know some people who are not very sensitive - they never get interference because it would be too much like hard work, especially when there are sensitive people like you around."

"That makes sense. I know a few people that wouldn't even know what sensitive means, so I can understand what you mean."

"Okay. Are you sure you're going to be alright tonight?"

"Yes, I just need to stay positive. I'm feeling much better now - thanks for talking to me."

"That's okay. Let me know if you need any more help. I'm only at the end of a phone. Good night."

"Thanks. Good night."

It wasn't until the following week that I spoke to Rose again. I had decided to phone her as I hadn't spoken to her for a few days, just to see how she was holding up.

"Hello, Rose. How are you getting on?"

"Oh I'm alright, but I can't talk now I'm not feeling well. I have a stomach ache and a headache that I just can't seem to shift. I'll be okay in a few days. Thanks for calling. Bye."

Rose had put the phone down. I didn't like the feelings I got while she was talking. She seemed very depressed and I knew the aches she was suffering weren't hers. I resolved to drop by her house in the morning, which was Saturday, to see for myself what was going on. The following morning I knocked on Rose's door and when she opened it I could see she was in trouble. There was a very heavy feeling of depression and her eyes were darting this way and that. She was looking very drawn and tired and it was easy to see she wasn't sleeping.

"Hello, Rose. I was passing and thought I would drop in to see how you were getting on. I was worried about you after we spoke last night."

Rose invited me in and sat on her armchair looking listless, as though she had given up on life. I was aware of an oppressive feeling and the house was very cold, although Rose didn't seem to notice.

"What's been happening, Rose?" I asked.

"Just the normal things. I have been going to work and coming home and studying and then going to bed and starting all over again the next day."

"How's your head and stomach? You were saying last night you've had pains in both your head and stomach for a few days."

"Oh they're OK. I've got used to it now, they'll go in a while."

I was aware of a man standing next to Rose and he didn't look very nice: he appeared to have surrounded her in a very unsettling energy. It was as though he was controlling her emotions. I decided if Rose would let me, that I would get rid of him and stop the pains he was giving her.

"If you like, I'll give you some healing. Maybe I can help you to get rid of your headache. Have you taken anything for it?"

"Yes, but they don't work. I've given up with the pills - nothing seems to work anymore."

"Have you seen the doctor?"

"Yes. They just say I'm run down and need to rest. I was going to spend the weekend in bed to try and shift this heavy feeling, but I can't sleep."

"As I'm here, would you like me to give you some healing and see if I can help?"

I knew what the problem was, but without Rose's permission there was nothing I could do. I wouldn't invade her space and I couldn't give her healing or do anything if she didn't want me to.

"Yes please, if you think it will help."

I asked Rose to sit on a chair, where she sat with shoulders drooped. I stood behind her and placed my hands on her shoulders. She flinched but stayed where she was and I could feel the man trying to attack me. I asked my guides to assist me, and together we removed him from her and placed him in a bubble of light. I continued to give Rose healing and gradually she straightened up. I focused on her head to start with and when I was comfortable that her head was OK, I then moved to her lower back.

"How did you know my back was hurting?" she asked.

"Because I could feel it, and I knew that your stomach was troubling you as well as your head. How do you feel now?" I said.

"My head feels better and my stomach and back pains are starting to go. What've you done?"

"I've just asked my guides to help me to remove a man that was giving you the pains. Now I'm helping your body to settle down after being invaded by him. You'll feel fine in a few minutes - just relax. How are you feeling now?"

"I'm feeling much better. Have I been attacked again? I thought it was just me."

"Yes, you've been in this house now for a week and gradually they've been undermining you and dragging you down. When I came in I noticed how heavy the atmosphere was - you probably never noticed because you've got used to it. They've been attacking you all the time you've been at home. Tell me, how has it been at work?"

"It's been the same as it always has, depressing, and everyone seems to get at me for no reason. At college I just can't seem to focus, I don't remember the lessons and when I try to study I don't have a clue what I'm supposed to be doing."

"You thought it was just you feeling under the weather, didn't you? They're very cunning; they will gently drag you down and isolate you, as they have done over the past week. It's no wonder you didn't want to talk to me. I suppose they've also convinced you that I'm evil and the cause of all your problems too?"

"Well yes, I felt you were causing me lots of aggravation because I didn't have so much trouble until you came to clear the house."

"The reason you're having more trouble is because you're fighting and winning, and they're trying to get you back under their thumb, so to speak. By leaving you here for the past week I was hoping I had set you on the road to getting rid of them. I can see now it was a mistake to leave you on your own so soon. That's my fault for letting you try to deal with it by yourself - you weren't ready. They've been very sneaky, but that's their nature. We'll have to go about this in a different way."

"It's my fault for not being vigilant enough and letting them get in. I'm sorry."

"There's no need to be sorry - you were attacked while you were asleep as well as during your waking hours. It's easy to make you think something if you wake up to those thoughts and you have no reference to what's normal. If you're up to it, let's take a walk and get you out of the house for a little while and give you a chance to settle down. "

"Well, I have a lot to do but I suppose half an hour won't hurt."

I knew once Rose was out of the house she would feel better, and it would be no good her trying to study feeling the way she was at the moment. We went down to the beach and I left her to gather her thoughts as we walked along in silence. After about ten minutes she seemed to brighten a bit. I said nothing, just giving her time to adjust. Then she said:

"Those bastards have been having it their own way for too long. It's plain to see I can't deal with them by myself at the moment - what am I going to do?"

"Well, as it's Saturday, if you like, you can come over to mine for the day and do your studying while I watch over your emotions and moods. If I sense a change then I'll warn you and together we can deal with it. I have things to do around the house, so I won't be sitting watching you, but it will give me a chance to observe and you a chance to get some studying done. What do you think?"

"I couldn't put you to so much trouble - you've done enough. It's up to me to sort this out now you've shown me the way."

"It's no trouble. I had no plans apart from pottering around the house so you wouldn't be in the way, and I don't like the way they're taking advantage of you - it's time it stopped. The only way I can see to stop it is to be there and warn you when they're attacking, so at least you have a chance to defend yourself. If you're unable to, then once I sort it out I can explain how to deal with it if it happens again."

"Well if you're sure ... I'll put some stuff together when we get back and meet you at your house."

"No, I'll wait for you in case you get attacked again while you're getting ready, then you can follow me back."

"Okay, let's get started."

Rose seemed to have perked up quite a bit and when we got back to her house she went round gathering up her books and study things, then got her coat and announced she was ready.

Suddenly it went very cold and Rose's eyes started to glaze over, I took her arm and led her out of the house, where she seemed to regain her composure.

"I'm sorry, I don't know what came over me. I just couldn't control what was happening - one minute I was angry, then I was sad and I couldn't stop it."

"Yes, they hit you with as much as they could to make your emotions go all over the place. If I had left you, they would have taken you over or made you angry at me, so we had to get out to stabilise the situation for you. Are you going to be alright to drive?"

"Yes, just give me a minute to sort myself out, then we can go."

Home

We arrived at my house without any problems and once Rose had settled herself in, she took out her study material and - armed with a cup of tea - got to work. I pottered round doing odd chores while Rose was working. I was passing through the lounge where Rose was and noticed a heavy atmosphere around her. I asked. "Are you alright?"

Rose looked up and said: "I've been sitting here for a while trying to remember what I'm supposed to be doing. I know I'm studying, but I can't concentrate and I keep making silly mistakes. I also don't like the window like that - people can see me and are watching. Can you close the curtains?"

The windows all have nets in them and in daylight it's not possible to see in, but I closed the curtains anyway to give Rose one less thing to worry about.

"Well, as you've been studying for about four hours I think it's time you had a break. Would you like to go for a walk?"

"Yes, maybe a change of surroundings will help me focus better."

We got ready and went out along the seafront. As we walked, I asked Rose: "Do you find that happens very often?"

"Yes. I also find when I go to college I can't take in what's being said. Sometimes I come home and haven't a clue what the tutor has said. It's very frustrating."

"When I came into the lounge I could feel a heavy presence around you, which is why I suggested a walk to change your energy."

"Was I being attacked again?"

"Yes, but it's not as obvious as before. They're trying to undermine your confidence in your ability to study so that you'll feel depressed because you can't remember what you're doing. It's another way of distracting you and driving you down into depression, so it's easier to control you."

"How do I fight it if I don't know when it's happening?"

"That's one of the reasons you're studying here, so I can keep an eye on you and deal with things as they arise. By changing your energy you should be feeling less confused and more alert now."

"Yes, I do feel better, but isn't that normal when you've been working to take a break to recharge your batteries?"

"Yes, but usually it's because you're feeling a bit tired or need to stretch. This is different because not only were you not feeling tired, but your mind was confused. By getting out of the room, you've removed yourself from the negative influences that were attacking you."

"But I can't keep going for a walk - what if I'm at work?"

"Let's take it one step at a time. First recognise you're being attacked, then we'll deal with it."

"How long is it going to take for me to recognise when I am being attacked?"

"Not long. Once you know what they're capable of you'll recognise it much sooner."

We returned home and Rose decided she would have another go at studying and managed quite well for about an hour, then she gave it a rest. We had something to eat and talked about how things were going.

Rose said: "There seems to be lots of ways the nasty spirits can attack me. How am I ever going to sort it out?"

"By me warning you or helping you to deal with the problems they give you, you'll start to recognise what's happening to you sooner, and that will make it easier for us and you to deal with it. For instance, how do you feel now?"

"I feel okay, not depressed or excited - just normal, I suppose."

"Remember how it feels and if you feel agitated or upset suddenly, then think about why you would feel that way. If nothing has happened to make you agitated, then it's not you. It can be very subtle, but with practice and by being alert, you'll notice the changes. When you do, change what you're doing and move about a bit."

"When you say change what you're doing, how do you mean?"

"Just go and make a cup of tea or speak to someone if you're in company, like at work or college. If you're on your own, just get up and go into another room or put some music on - anything to change your thought process, even if it's just for a short while. While you're doing that, think about what's been happening and you'll realise it isn't you. Because you're particularly sensitive and these things have been attacking you for so long it's easy for them to influence you. By analysing what thoughts are going through your head you'll start to recognise the stray ones - ones not connected to what you're doing. Usually when someone joins a development circle we try to help them recognise what is and isn't their thoughts. They then know when spirit is communicating with them, but in your case you're already getting it - it's just a case of knowing when."

"Do you mean like psychic readings?"

"Not quite. You see, when you're doing psychic readings you'll be tuning in to the aura of your sitter and in the beginning you won't know what's psychic and what's spirit. With guidance from the circle leader you'll learn to tell the difference. For instance, you may be talking about feelings you're picking up from someone and suddenly you'll say they had a disagreement with somebody yesterday or something like that. You won't pick up information like that in a psychic reading - someone from spirit is telling you. It's little things like that which will help the developing medium to recognise their thoughts and spirit communication. In your case, you've been getting spirit communication for a long time and it's become second-nature to you. You think it's your own thoughts, so we have to work in a different way to help you recognise the difference. We have to look at all your thoughts and put them into perspective for you. Take now, for instance - you know there's someone listening and you know exactly where they are, don't you?"

"Yes, I didn't think you'd noticed. What do they want?"

"They're just waiting for a chance to attack you, but now we've spoken about them they won't bother, because they know we're ready for them. They only attack when they think they won't be noticed. The whole idea is to make you think you're, as you put it, a nut job - that's where they get their fun. If you know it's them, there's no fun in it so there's no point. You see you're calming down again now - you know they're not going to attack. Did you notice how you started to tense up? That's because, deep down in your subconscious, you recognise when they're around you. All we have to do is bring that recognition to the conscious mind. You also keep getting this feeling of being watched: that's also spirit. The neighbours can't see in with the nets there unless it's dark and the lights are on."

"So I do know what's going on, but because I've got used to it, I don't recognise it as easily as you do."

"Yes, that's right, but with a little bit of work and time we should be able to get you back on track."

"So once I start to recognise what's happening then I have to stop it. That's not going to be easy - I've tried before and failed."

"That's not true. Earlier this afternoon you stopped an attack when we went for a walk."

Rose's face brightened. "Yes I did, so it's that easy, is it?"

"Sometimes if you recognise it soon enough, but if they get into your mind, then it can be quite a fight to get things under your control again."

Rose decided to do some more studying as it was still early, so I left her to it while I tidied up and then sat and read a book so I could keep a close eye on her.

After about an hour Rose got up, saying she'd had enough for today, so she gathered her things together and took them out to her car. She came back and thanked me and then she went home. I asked her to call me before she went to bed so I'd know she was OK.

Rose called and said she had watched a couple of comedy programmes when she got home and now she was feeling tired and was going to bed. She said she was a bit worried about going to bed.

"What are you afraid of?"

"Well it's dark and this is usually the time I get the worst attacks."

"Do you remember what I said about fear breeding fear? Well this is one of those times - there is nothing to fear. They're cowards and if you confront them they'll go away. Have faith in yourself and ask your guides to protect you."

"But I don't know any guides."

"It doesn't matter. They know you and can hear what you're saying and thinking - they will not let you get anything you can't handle."

"If that's true, then why have I suffered for so long with all the trouble I've had?"

"Although you may not know it, what you've gone through is part of your life's journey, and now it's time to get control of

163

things so you can move forward again."

"I don't feel like I've moved forward at all at the moment."

"Give yourself time. You've only just started on this part of your learning. It's all in there - we just have to bring it to the front of your mind. Now why don't you close yourself down like we've practised?"

" I'll give it a try."

"You have to be more positive than that. Remember, it's your intention that makes it work, so have confidence and trust in your guides. Sometimes they may allow a little to get in just to teach you, but they know what they're doing as they look at the longer term, not just the now."

Rose went through her routine, setting up her protection and closing down, and when she had finished she said:

"That's done and I didn't have any problems this time."

"Good. Call me if you have any problems, although I'm sure you will be able to handle it if anything happens."

Just as I was hanging up, Rose cried out.

"What happened? I asked.

"Somebody jumped out at me and made me jump. I thought you said the protection would work."

"You didn't get taken over, did you? So you were surprised because someone jumped out at you, but you're OK now, aren't you?"

"Well, yes. I suppose it's quite funny really jumping at shadows, although it wasn't a shadow - there was someone there."

"Yes, but you know there are spirits around us all the time. Why should you be surprised that you saw one? You've been seeing them all your life."

"Yes, I just wasn't expecting it to happen then. Right, I'm going to bed now. Good night."

"Don't forget to do your visualisation while you're waiting to drop off to sleep - it will keep your mind under control."

"Do I need to do it every night?"

"For the time being. It won't hurt and you'll be learning mind control."

I said goodnight and put the phone down. The next morning Rose called me and said:

"I had an interesting night, to say the least. It started when I closed my eyes. I saw faces, so I did what you said and opened my eyes. When I closed my eyes again they came back, so I sat up and waited for about ten minutes. As I was trying to go to sleep again I kept getting very hot, so I opened my eyes and when I closed them I started getting cold. When I opened my eyes again that went away and so I focused on closing down and that's the last I knew until I woke up this morning."

"You did well then. You should be proud of yourself - you managed to counteract everything they threw at you and go to sleep."

"I see. Does that mean I'm getting on top of this?"

"It's part of the process, a little bit at a time, but you're moving in the right direction. You will have some setbacks, but don't give up on yourself - you're doing very well."

"I did wake up at one time but I couldn't move. I started to panic, then it just went away and I went back to sleep. I was so tired."

"Yes, that happens sometimes. It's where spirit control your movements and your ability to speak."

"Why do they do that to people? What's the point? Is it so they can possess them or just to upset them?"

"Well, it's a bit of both. By upsetting you they're helping others get you under their control, and by controlling your movements and your ability to speak, it is if you like, a precursor to possession."

"Why don't they possess the insensitive people. Surely that would be easier?"

"They do. There are lots of people on medication and in institutions who are taken over by spirit, but because of the strong medication it's not recognised for what it is. You have to remember why they attack people. To put it all in perspective, there's no point in controlling someone who's not aware they're being controlled, except for practice. There are no brownie points to be gained. If, on the other hand, they can control a sensitive person who fights back, then they gain more respect from their peers. They have nothing else to do but prey on the weak or unaware. They do it because they're bullies and cowards. If they weren't cowards they would attack mediums, who are more aware and can defend themselves."

165

"Have you ever been attacked like that?"

"No but my ex was on a number of occasions, until we understood what was going on and managed to overcome it."

"How did you find out what was going on?"

"We were fortunate that my ex went into light trance, so I was able to ask one of her guides about it. He explained what was happening and how to overcome it and after a few tries we managed it."

"How did you overcome it?"

"First I had to tune in to my ex, so that when I was asleep I would be aware of her. When she was attacked she would go stiff and moan like she was dreaming. I would wake her up by gently and call her name while holding her hand to ground her. She had to relax and talk to her guides when she was aware of it happening. She found it easier to get it under control by not panicking, just calmly talking to her guides about what was happening. The spirit who was attacking her was aware of what she was doing, and because she was no longer panicking, there became no point in continuing the attacks. In that way we were able to gradually get things under control. It took about three weeks but she was only attacked a few times a week."

"So if it happens to me again, I just lie there, relax and talk to my guides, and it will stop?"

"Why don't you try it if it happens again? You won't stop it on your first go, but gradually it will stop - the trick is to recognise it when it happens. Now it's getting late, so I suggest you lie down on the sofa as you're not keen on going back to bed, and try to get some more sleep. One of the hardest things to fight is tiredness and the more tired you get, the easier it is for the nasty spirits to interfere. It's also another way they will attack, by making you feel tired. That's why it's so important to monitor the amount of sleep you get, then you'll know whether you should be tired or not."

Rose came back to do some more studying and about midday I asked:

"Have you felt anything this morning?"

"Not really. I thought you walked through the room a couple of times, but it wasn't you, as when I saw you next, you came from the wrong direction, so I must have been aware of spirit moving about. I managed to ignore it and focused on what I was doing and things seemed to be alright."

Rose seemed more at ease as she settled down again to study, saying it was much more peaceful than at home, and she felt safer with someone watching over her. I didn't want her to become dependent on me as she would never gain the confidence to fight when she was on her own, so I decided to go out for a while and leave her to study. I told her to help herself to whatever she wanted and that I wouldn't be long, and went off to the shops.

I was gone about two hours and when I got back Rose was busy working, so I didn't interrupt. She seemed OK and I wasn't aware of anything interfering with her, so I went out into the garden to do a few little jobs. While I was out there, I felt a presence and when I looked up, Rose was standing drinking a cup of tea. She looked calm and in control and I asked her:

"How's it going? No problems?"

"No, this afternoon seems to be going fine. I was a bit worried when you went to the shop but soon settled down. I've managed to do all my work - don't know if it's right, we'll have to see."

"Well it was worth coming over again to do it then, wasn't it?"

"Yes I'm going to pack up my things as I have to get a few things done before I go to bed tonight."

"Right. I've nearly finished what I'm doing and I'll see you off."

Once Rose had packed her things and put them in her car, she came and thanked me for my help and I told her:

"Be aware and don't let yourself get upset or depressed. If you have another attack, just deal with it as best you can, and try to stay peaceful."

"I'm feeling a bit more confident at the moment. I know I'll be alright. As you said, it just takes a little while to understand what's going on. Right, I'm off. I'll talk to you later."

"Yes, just let me know you're okay before you go to bed."

"Okay, bye for now."

As I watched her go I wondered if she would get any problems that night. I felt if she did she would be able to sort them out, if she thought about things before she acted.

It was about ten when Rose phoned and I asked her:

"How are things at home?"

"It's a bit depressing so I'm watching a bit of television and chilling before I go to bed. I'm okay. I can feel things but I'm ignoring them. I haven't had anything major happen."

"Try and forget all about it. I know it's easier said than done, but the less you think about it, the less it will affect you. Take care and call me when you get in from work so I know you're alright. It's not over yet, but the more you get things under control, the less you'll be bothered."

"Alright. Thanks again - speak to you tomorrow."

At Work

Rose phoned about ten in the morning and I could hear the distress in her voice.

I asked: "How are you?"

"I'm having problems. I came to work feeling fine. I had a few problems during the night but managed to overcome them, but today when I got to work it started to go downhill. I sit opposite a lady who is around 60 and she can be very negative. I was alright until she came in and then things just got worse. It's like she brings negative spirits with her and unloads them onto me."

"One of the problems is your sensitivity - you pick up negative influences. Unlike most people who just ignore them and get on with things, you tend to focus on them and draw them to you. You empathise too much, and take on board the feelings she's experiencing, and make them your own. You need to get a thicker skin and not allow her to unload on you. I bet she's feeling better now, isn't she?"

"She seems to be as cheerful as she ever gets. I guess it's true - do you mean she does it on purpose?"

"She may not know what she's doing, but there are lots of people like her. The trick is to listen, but then to let it go. I bet you're feeling sorry for her and thinking about what she's told you, aren't you?"

"Yes I suppose I am. How do I get rid of these feelings?"

"Well the first thing is to stop feeling sorry for her and let it go - it's not your problem."

"But it's like she's sending negative things to me even when she isn't saying anything."

"Yes, that's what you're picking up because you're open to other people's feelings. You have to close yourself down and protect yourself. Go for a break and when you come back try putting an imaginary wall up between you. Then smile and get on with what you have to do and ignore the vibes you're getting from her direction."

"Why is she doing this to me?"

"She probably doesn't know what she's doing - it's most likely the way she is. It's you that has to learn to control what you pick up. I doubt she's the only one that makes you feel the way you are.

There are lots like her, and not many like you. Believe me when I tell you there are those who know how to unload their problems and walk away feeling better, while the person they have unloaded to is feeling quite low. They're like leeches sometimes - they suck all the good vibrations from you and leave theirs behind for you to pick up. I bet when you go to a hospital, you feel drained when you leave, don't you?"

"Yes I do and I get irritated. Why does that happen?"

"In a hospital there are a lot of unhappy people who are suffering, you just zero in on their feelings and it drains you. You can't help everyone - they also have their lessons to learn. No matter how much you want to help everyone you can't, because they have to learn for themselves. Most people are able to put these feelings aside and get on with things, but I'm sure you've met others who feel drained when they listen to other people's problems. I know you don't do it on purpose, but you need to recognise what's going on, so you can protect yourself. Once you stop drawing in their negativity you'll feel much better. You'll be able to keep your emotions level, which will make it harder for bad spirits to gain a hold over you. I'll bet you've been getting other feelings, about being watched, or feeling as though nobody likes you, and wanting to give up on everything. It's just another way of spirit making use of the opportunity you're giving them to get at you."

"I see what you mean. It's as though I'm on a roller-coaster, going downhill with my feelings, and it all started when she got here. How am I going to stop it?"

"Think about what I've said - don't blame yourself, but do what I suggested. Change your energy and come back to your desk with a positive outlook. If necessary ask your guides to help get rid of the negativity, trust that they will and then forget about it and move on."

"I'll do that. Thanks for listening, I'll call you later and let you know how I'm getting on."

Later that day Rose phoned:

"Hi. I managed to get past this morning by doing what you said. I didn't manage it straight away, but after a while I realised I was feeling better. I'm home now and when I came in it was like walking into a wall of misery, so I put some music on and have been singing along to try to raise my vibrations. It worked for a while but gradually I've been sinking into that misery. I'm okay, just starting to feel a bit down. I'm just about to do some studying ready for college tomorrow night."

"That's good. Stay positive and remember it's you that changes how things are by not accepting negativity. If you're feeling negative, ask yourself why all of a sudden you feel that way. Think about what's happened to change how you're feeling - if there's nothing obvious, then it's not you and say so out loud. Let the nasty spirits know that you recognise what they're doing and refuse to accept it. You'll be surprised at how quickly your mood changes for the better if you can stay positive. Try not to get angry, but be determined that you're not going to allow them to manipulate you. Don't forget to ask for protection and close yourself down before you go to bed."

"I'm finding closing down isn't helping much. I just seem to get aggravation anyway. Is there anything else I can do to protect myself? Maybe I can do an angel meditation - I always felt better when I did that. What do you think?"

"If it makes you feel good, do it. There's more than one way to protect yourself, so do what suits you best. I know how you feel about angels and crystals, so why don't you combine the two? It's not about what you do that makes it work - it's about what you believe in. Enjoy your evening and call if you need me."

"Hopefully I'll be okay. Talk to you later."

I spoke to Rose the following day at work and she said.

"When Jackie, the women that sits opposite me, came in today, I was ready for her. I just said 'good morning' and smiled, then got on with my work. I started picking up a prickly feeling around her, so I just sent her love and light and then ignored her. So far I'm doing alright - although there are negative feelings around, I'm managing to keep them at bay. I think my angel meditation might have something to do with it. Anyway, I'm staying positive and hopefully things will be alright. I'm a bit tired, as I had a restless night, but otherwise okay."

"Good - so your angel meditation is working for you. It's as I said, it's what you believe that makes it work. Have a good day and I'll talk to you soon."

Over the next few months Rose progressed and managed to get things under her control. She had the occasional relapse, but generally has progressed to such an extent she is now sitting in a development circle and making use of her ability as a clairvoyant. She is giving very good evidence and her messages are understood by the recipients. She sometimes gets interference during her circle work and we talk it through, and sort out what happened, so she will be aware of it next time. She's staying positive and her whole outlook has changed. She's much calmer and less inclined to believe people are against her, or that she's being watched. All in all, a well-balanced person with a lot more self-belief and confidence.

Rose still gets the occasional attack, about once a week, and because they are so much more subtle they can take longer to notice. They're not so intense, but because it takes a while to recognise: they tend to drag her further down before she realises what's happening. Once she realises, then she removes the troublesome spirits and she's fine again. The trick now is to recognise her own moods and know when it's Rose, or outside influences.

Over the next few months Rose progressed to such an extent she now has much more control over any interference she gets. Not only is she able to recognise when she is being attacked, but she has been able to see when others are being influenced.

After about six months, Rose asked if it would be alright to start her healing again as I'd said she shouldn't do it until she had things under control.

I said that should be okay and over the past years she has gone from strength to strength. Because of Rose's experience, she is an invaluable source of knowledge and understanding. When she talks to people she is able to empathise with them and help them understand.

This case took about two years to resolve, which shows what a difficult job it can be for someone in the middle of all that negativity. It also shows how much courage and determination is required to beat spirit interference sometimes. Not all cases take so long: it just depends on when we are able to start the process and on the intensity and determination of the attacks from the spirit world.

Case 3

It was in March 2013 that were received a telephone call from a woman called Miriam. She said she was a carer for a woman called Toni who was having a lot of spiritual activity at her flat. When I asked her what kind of activity she replied:

"Toni keeps having her furniture moved and is experiencing electrical problems. Her cooker keeps getting turned on, as does her washing machine. If she wants to use the cooker she has to keep an eye on it because sometimes it gets turned off again. One day she took her dogs for a walk, and when she came back the cold water tap was turned full on - fortunately she wasn't flooded. Toni now turns it off at the mains when she's not using it. When she comes home after shopping or just going out, she finds all the drawers and doors to her kitchen cupboards have been opened; the fridge and freezer doors are also opened. She has trouble sleeping and concentrating on anything for very long. She's had to store all her furniture in the bedrooms and lock the doors, for fear of something being pushed onto her while she's sleeping. She has a mattress in the lounge where she sleeps, so she can keep an eye on the kitchen. Her smoke alarm goes off for no reason and she can't take the batteries out because it's run off the mains. Is there anything you can do to help?"

"Can you tell me what's wrong with her, and has she had the electrics checked?"

Miriam replied: "To start at the beginning, when she was little she was sexually abused by her father, but her mother and gran just ignored her when she told them. They told her to stop making up wicked lies. That continued until she was 16 when she left home and was living on the streets. During her childhood she was getting voices in her head, telling her things about people that were private. If she told anyone they would chastise her for telling lies. Her gran told her she was evil and kept taking her to the Catholic Church. The priest would tell her off and make her say prayers for forgiveness. In the end he gave up on her and told her gran not to bring her back. You can imagine how a little girl of seven would feel when she's told not to come back to the church. Toni, since she left home, has been married once, but that didn't last and now at 25 she is living in sheltered housing. In the last eight years she has had to move four times because of trouble in her flat from spirit activity, but it keeps following her."

"Do you know if she has ever used the Ouija board or dabbled with the occult?"

"Yes she used to use the Ouija board a lot in one flat, but the activity got so bad she stopped and moved. She's also been involved with witchcraft and Satanism, because she had a pentagon engraved on the walls in the flat before this one. That's why she had to move the last time, to try and get away from it. She has also been involved in wicca to try and stop the spiritual activity, by casting spells to neutralise the bad energies. At the moment she has a spirit which we call Canute who likes to play games with her. If she doesn't play, then he gets nasty and throws things around. Sometimes he follows me home because I'm a bit psychic. I am aware of him and he causes trouble at my house. Toni was diagnosed with schizophrenia about four years ago and has been on medication ever since, but it's not making any difference. When she went to the psychiatrist recently they changed her diagnosis to split personality. Since her gran died, Toni has been haunted by her. Her gran says she hates her - I've actually heard her say it."

"Wow, she's certainly been busy. Although we're willing to come and clear the spirits from her flat, I fear we won't be able to keep it clear, unless Toni realises that there will be a lot of work to do to stop it coming back. We are mediums not psychiatrists, so although we can deal with the spirits, it'll be a long uphill battle for Toni to get control of her situation. We will guide her and help her but it will take quite a long time - it's not a quick fix."

"When you say a long time, how long will it take?"

"That really depends on Toni. She'll have to do all the work. We can teach her and support her, but it's got to come from her. A year, maybe two, but it's going to be constant fighting every day and once she starts, she can't give up or she'll go straight back to where she started. We can't tell her to stop taking her medication, so it may be difficult for her. What we do is teach her to control the thoughts that she gets and help her to train her mind so she can block the interference she is getting. She has to start taking responsibility for what goes on around her. Do you think she can do that?"

"I don't know. I thought you would just come and clear it and that would be it."

"We've only talked about schizophrenia, where she is hearing voices. If they are now saying she has split personality disorder that would be a whole new ball game. If she has split personalities, then is she aware of them and does she know when they're there and can she control them?"

"She's been told by the psychiatrist that she's got about 20 with her. She knows some of them - that's all I know."

"From what you've said it would appear the furniture is being moved by Toni when she is in an altered state that she is not aware of. When it goes, she thinks it's been done by spirit."

"When you say altered state, do you mean she's taken over by spirit?"

"Yes. You see if she has a number of spirits taking control of her consciousness at different times, her memory will have gaps when they were in control. Because she has no memory of doing things at these times, she is going to think it's discarnate spirit who are doing it. This would explain the furniture and the tap and also the cooker and fridge and the cupboard doors and drawers being opened."

"So you're saying she's doing it when she's got one of alters with her. Is there anything you can do?"

"I think we should come and see her. I just thought I should make you aware of the possibilities. At least we can clear what's there and then assess the situation. We can then talk to Toni about the way forward and what it will entail."

"Okay, when will you be able to come?"

"I'll get back to you when I've arranged things with the rest of the team. I assume evening would be okay?"

"Yes, any evening. I'll meet you there - just let me know."

Talking to Vanessa and Danny, I explained the situation and after I had described what Miriam had told me, we all agreed it seemed like Toni had what is termed as undifferentiated schizophrenia, schizoaffective disorder and MPD which are described as:-

Undifferentiated schizophrenia:

Conditions meeting the general diagnostic criteria for schizophrenia but not conforming to any of the other subtypes. Or exhibiting the features of more than one of them, without a clear predominance of a particular set of diagnostic characteristics.

Schizoaffective disorder:

These people have symptoms of schizophrenia as well as mood disorder such as major depression, bipolar mania or mixed mania.

Multiple Personality Disorder:

This is where an individual has more than one spirit around them who takes control of the consciousness. When this happens they are doing things which only logs in the spirits' consciousness and the individual has no recollection of what's taken place. When the individual get a number of alters interfering with their daily life, the timeline of the memory will get fragmented. It's no wonder people think they are losing their mind.

These appear to be the clinical definitions of Toni's condition. We decided to go and see if we could help. Even if we were only able to clear the current problem, we would be able to explain to Toni what she would have to do and how we would support her. I called Miriam to let her know when we were able to come along.

On arrival we found that Toni lived in a flat on the first floor at the back of the building. We buzzed the front door and Toni let us in, then we knocked on her flat door and, after telling her who we were, she let us in, saying Miriam would be about five minutes. She invited us in while trying to calm her dogs. We all made friends with the dogs and they settled down and we went into the lounge. There was a mattress on the floor with a television beside it. There was also a tall cupboard which was laid on its back on the other side of the lounge. It was a lounge-diner and although the kitchen was respectable, the lounge floor had lino on it. It was quite wet in places where the dogs had been unable to hold on. We sat on the window-sill as there was no-where else and chatted to Toni about her problems as we waited for Miriam.

"Hi Toni. This is Vanessa and Danny and I'm Mike. We've had a chat with Miriam and she's told us about your situation. I would like to ask you a few questions while we're waiting for her, if that's okay. We are not medically trained - we are mediums who deal with spirits that interfere with people's lives."

"Yes - what would you like to know?"

"Have you always been able to hear voices in your head?"

"Yes. Sometimes I have a conversation with them and usually I don't remember what happens next. It's as though I've been to sleep for a while or something, because I've often found myself in another room when I've come to. Did Miriam tell you about the kitchen cupboards? Quite often all the drawers are open and the doors too. I think spirit keep opening them to annoy me. They also keep ringing the front door bell and the flat bell as well. The other night it went on for most of the night."

"Okay, we're going to tell you what we can do and what we can't. We'll also explain how we can help you and with Miriam's help we may be able to resolve some of your problems."

Just then the doorbell rang and Toni let Miriam in. She was accompanied by her husband Ray and after the introductions we explained how we would be able to help.

"Now, Miriam has told us about your condition. It's going to be a long fight and you're going to have to be strong and determined. Once we start there is no turning back, because to do so will put you right back at the start. We can clear the current spirits in the flat, but you're going to have to learn how to control your mind and focus on the positive. We'll show you what to do and teach you how, and we'll also be there for you 24/7 if you need to talk or need advice. We would need to come here at least once a week in the first instance to make sure you're still clear, or to clear any spirits that have come in during the week. Make no mistake - it's not a quick fix . It's going to be hard and it could take a year or more. I will tell you now that schizophrenia is a complaint that has never been cured by drugs. In fact many people have been able to overcome it without drugs - it's called milieu therapy. Most either come to terms with it, or it goes away after about five years - sometimes more, sometimes less. Tell me - are you on any medication for your condition?"

"Yes, I'm on quite a few. Miriam helps me to sort them out each day."

Toni showed us a large bag which was full of different medications.

"How long have you been taking these?" Vanessa asked.

"For about 10 years. It got so bad that my mum and gran took me to see the doctor. He sent me to a psychiatrist who prescribed the pills. He changes them every now and then, depending on how I'm feeling."

"Hopefully he will see the changes in you and maybe reduce them for you. We can't tell you what to do about your medication - that will have to be up to the psychiatrist. But if we can help you to come to terms and deal with what's going on around you, then he may reduce your medication over a time as you become more able to cope. You see the medication can have an effect on your brain, we'll never know. But let's look on the positive side. First we'll clear the spirits that are here now, then we'll see what's next."

Vanessa told us about a spirit who she was aware of in the lounge and Danny brought her through. She wasn't very nice, but after some discussion we managed to persuade her to go to her family. Then we picked up a nasty man who had been giving Toni pains in her head and stomach and who saw the error of his ways and went to the light. After we had dealt with about 10 spirits, we came across an old lady whose description matched Toni's gran, much to our surprise. She was adamant she was going no-where until we showed her where her mother was and her sisters. She then, without apology, asked to be allowed to join them, which we allowed her to do, because it was one less to annoy Toni, and we didn't want to send anyone out into the dark. Toni felt much better after she had gone, so we focused on her and this is what happened.

"Danny, can you give Toni some healing?" I asked.

"Yes okay," he said as he went and brought an armchair in from one of the bedrooms, after asking if it would be alright to do so. As I said, there was no furniture in the lounge - it was all stacked up in the two bedrooms.

"Why is the furniture in the bedrooms?" I asked.

"When I go out, sometimes when I come home, the lounge door won't open because someone's pushed an armchair up against it and I can't get in. Ray has to come round and help me. Sometimes the furniture gets moved around when I'm here and I don't want the dogs getting hurt, so I lock it in the bedrooms," Toni said.

"Oh I see," I said.

Danny went round the back of the armchair and placed his hands on Toni's shoulders, so that he could sense if Toni had any attachments with her. He looked at me and nodded. Both Vanessa and I went to help him. Vanessa asked if she could place her hands on Toni's throat chakra and solar plexus to help Danny remove the attachments, while I stood ready to talk to any spirits if Toni was possessed.

Toni sat there for a moment and then her eyes rolled up into her head and she started shaking. I took her hand after telling her I was going to, and addressed the spirit who was with her.

"Hello, what are you doing here?"

The voice that came out of Toni's mouth was more like an old woman's than Toni's.

"She's mine now. Go away and leave us alone. Don't meddle in things you don't understand."

"How can she be yours? You don't own her. Toni has a life to lead in her own way. Why are you causing her so much trouble, and how did you attach yourself to her?"

"She came over here and when we saw she was going back, we just came with her. Now leave us in peace."

"I'm sorry we can't do that. You're obviously troubled if you think what you're doing is right."

"So, what do you think you're going to do about it, as if you could do anything anyway?"

"We're going to help you to go and be with you family where you belong. They're in heaven, you know - shall we take you to see them?"

"There's no such place. I know I've looked. This is nice and cosy here and I'm not leaving on your say so. You just want me to let her go - you don't care what happens after that."

"We're going to take you into the light so you can see for yourself. If you really don't like it, then we won't leave you there. Can you feel it getting warmer? Why don't you open your eyes and have a look? I can see your family coming to meet you. Can you?"

"It's a trick. I can see some people who look familiar, but I don't believe you."

"That's okay. Just hold your arm out and tell me what you feel."

"I can feel someone holding my hand. It feels warm and gentle and I feel very calm all of a sudden. Is it really true that there's a heaven?"

"Yes and you're there now. Can you see your family?"

"Yes we're all together now. Thank you. I would never have believed it."

With that she went and gradually Toni's face slackened and she opened her eyes.

"There's more here you know," Toni said.

"Yes we know. We can only remove a few this time, otherwise you'll feel empty and uncomfortable. We have to do it a little at a time so you can adjust to the changes. From what the woman said, it would appear that you've died at least once and been brought back - is that right?"

"I have tried to commit suicide on a number of occasions with drugs and I jumped off a bridge once too. They say I died from an overdose on two occasions and they brought me back."

"Yes, you also brought some attachments who don't want to let go. They're also taking over your body in the form of possession it seems, as and when they feel like it. I think it's during those times that one or more of your alter egos is moving things and opening the drawers and cupboards. Of course when Toni comes back, you won't remember what's happened and because there's so much spirit activity, you think its spirit that's doing it."

"Are you saying I'm moving things myself but I don't remember because someone's taken me over?"

"Yes, you're not conscious of what you do while under their influence, so it's quite a surprise when you're again conscious of your surroundings. Like I said, it's not going to be easy and there is no quick fix. It's going to take time and hard work - are you going to be able to manage?"

"What's the alternative?"

"To carry on as you have been. If you start this you must finish it, or you'll just go back to how it's been," Vanessa said.

"Can you tell me what I've got to do?"

"You're going to have to learn how to control your mind and stop the attachments from taking you over. We'll teach you a meditation to help you and we'll also help you to understand what is spirit and what's you or your alter. We'll be back every week to talk to you and assess how things are going and clear anything that's too much for you. We'll also be on the end of the phone to talk you through things, so you understand what's happening whenever you need it. It's going to be a long journey. Are you up to it?" Vanessa said.

"I don't know. Can I think about it?"

"Yes of course, but the longer you leave it, the harder it'll be. Why don't you have a chat with Miriam and Ray, because they will be supporting you too as they're around you a lot, and see what they think? There's not much more we can do tonight as we've cleared the flat and removed some attachments. We need to let you settle down now before we do any more," said Vanessa.

It had taken four hours to get to this stage and we knew there was a lot more work to do. We said our goodbyes and left after making arrangements to come back in a couple of days.

On our way home, Danny said:

"You know, when you were talking to the spirits that had attached themselves to Toni, I was aware of quite a few being pulled off her by my guides. They were real nasty and didn't want to go. I felt they were attached to the ones you were talking to."

"That makes sense. They did seem to calm down fairly quickly after a few minutes and I did notice how much lighter it was around Toni when we'd finished," I said.

"What do you think - will she have the strength to fight this?" Danny said.

"We have to remember she's had it most of her life. It's going to be very hard for her to let go. I hope so, but we'll have to wait and see," Vanessa said.

I spoke to Miriam the following day and asked whether she thought Toni would be able to handle it.

"We talked to her and I don't think she quite understands what she's going to have to do. I'm not sure - she seems to like the company, even though she has a lot of trouble. She did ask me if I would go to the psychiatrist with her on her next appointment next week to see what he thought. I said I would, but I don't think he's going to understand what's going on. Otherwise he would have done something by now instead of feeding her pills. She didn't seem too happy about that, but she said she'd talk to you tomorrow night when you go round," said Miriam.

"We'll see you tomorrow night then. Thanks. Bye."

When we got to Toni's flat, Miriam and Ray were already there. They had some more chairs out, so we sat down and I asked Toni how things had been.

"After you left it was a lot quieter and I managed to get to sleep alright. During the night I was woken up a couple of times. I think I heard a noise. I had some bad dreams, but other than that it wasn't too bad. The next day, yesterday, things started happening - the dogs started barking at that corner but there was nothing to see. I had to go to the shops and when I came back the drawers and doors in the kitchen were all open again. Last night it took me about three hours to cook my dinner as the cooker kept getting turned off. Today it's been about the same with the doorbell keep ringing and the smoke alarm going off when there was no smoke."

"We're aware of a few spirits around the flat and you have something hanging round you. We'll clear the flat first and then have a look at what's with you. Is that alright? Then Vanessa will show you how to do a meditation to help you to start getting control of your mind."

"Is there a little fat man here?"

"Do you mean the one with the limp?" I asked.

"Yes, he's been annoying the dogs. Can you get rid of him?"

"If you can bring him through, Danny, we'll have a word with him and see if we can help."

"Hello. Are you alright? You seem to be a bit lost."

"I would be alright if those damned dogs would stop barking at me. I don't like dogs - they're dangerous."

"They're just protecting their territory. What're you doing here?"

"I'm trying to keep warm and out of everyone's way. She's got some nasty people around her, you know."

"Yes we know - that's why we're here, to help her to get rid of them. Now what about you? You aren't in the right place, you know - you don't have to stay here."

"What do you suggest, that I go to heaven? I know, I've heard others talking about it. They didn't believe it, why should I?"

"They do when we show them what was waiting for them. Would you like me to show you?"

"Really, and what do you show them?"

"I take them to meet their friends and family. Can you feel the warmth around you?"

183

"Yes, I wondered what that was. What are you doing?"

"We're taking you to heaven where you'll be able to be with Geraldine."

"If that were true, why haven't I seen her before?"

"Well if you open your eyes you will see her."

"It's a bit bright. Wait a minute - there she is. How did you do that?"

"It doesn't really matter, does it? You're home now - do you want to stay?"

"Of course I do. At least there are no dogs here. Thanks. Bye."

He was gone and after we cleared a few others we asked Toni whether she thought she was ready to start sorting things out.

"I've been thinking about what Vanessa said and I think if you can get rid of some more attachments, I might be able to focus on what I've got to do."

"Let's start by removing the one who calls himself Barry - he feels like he thinks he owns you. Just sit quietly and Danny will stand behind you while Vanessa gives you healing."

As we were preparing, Toni just rolled her eyes back and disappeared. The look that came over her face was pure hate.

"Hello. You're Barry, aren't you? Why are you causing so much grief for the lady?"

"You nosey old bastard - what's it got to do with you? She's mine and I'll do what I want."

"You have to leave. You don't belong here. We'll help you - if you want, you can go to heaven."

"You got to be joking. With what I've got here, I'm not going anywhere." he shouted.

Vanessa started saying the serenity prayer and he started to shout over her, saying:

"My god is stronger than yours ..." Vanessa changed to the Lord's Prayer after Barry started to recite it backwards. She just kept saying it over and over while he tried to shout her down. Toni was shaking and trying to punch us and kick us and then all of a sudden Barry stopped and hung his head.

"I've got him now - he's surrounded in light. What do you want me to do with him?" asked Danny.

184

"If you watch you'll see some of our guides coming forward to take him. I know he's fighting but he can't win."

Toni's face cleared and she opened her eyes.

"God, that was awful. I hope he's gone now."

"Yes, he's been taking you over for a long time. I think you picked him up when you were doing the Ouija board. How are you feeling?"

"I feel exhausted. Are there anymore?"

"We're just going to remove a couple more. I think there's a lady with you who can't talk, do you know about her?"

"I know about her," said Miriam. "Sometimes when I'm here she comes through and Toni just sits there doing and saying nothing. I've tried to talk to her, but in the end I wait for her to go and make sure Toni is alright before I leave."

"We'll give you a few minutes to settle down and then we'll have a chat with her. Don't let anyone take you off until I say so. I know there's someone trying to take you now, but I want you to fight it. It's your chance to show them you're not as easy to control as you were, and you're starting to control them."

Vanessa talked Toni through a meditation where she could visualise a pathway and showed her how to make it real in her mind. Toni couldn't focus, so Vanessa asked her to picture a matchstick and try to make it stay in her mind. She couldn't do that either. In the end we had to get her to look out of the window and watch the trees, then close her eyes while she was watching the trees and still see them. She managed to do that briefly and Vanessa told her to practise it until she could hold the picture in her mind for about a minute.

"We won't take you any further with that until you can hold it for a while, then we'll go to the next stage. If we take it in little steps, you'll soon get the hang of it," Vanessa said.

We gave Toni a few minutes to compose herself again after trying the meditation, then we asked her to let the woman through. As the woman came forward I was aware of her standing beside Toni and then Toni's eyes rolled up and she was there.

"I'm going to talk to you and all you have to do is nod or shake your head, okay?"

Nod.

"Do you know where you are?"

Nod.

"Do you know what's happened to you?"

Nod.

"Then you know you are able to speak now - the problem was with your physical body, not your spirit."

"I haven't tried to speak before in case I couldn't. It feels strange."

"You will get used to it, although you only have to think now and you will be heard. Would you like to go to heaven and be with your mother?"

"Yes please."

"Open your eyes and tell me if you can see something different. I'll be seeing what you see."

"I can see a beautiful light in front of me."

"We're going to go into that light - that's where your mother and father are, that's heaven, okay?"

"Yes - can we go now?"

"Take my hand and come with me; can you see them now?"

"Yes I can see a lot of my family."

"You can stay with them if you want to. You'll soon settle down. Do you want to stay?"

"Yes and thank you for everything - bless you."

Toni opened her eyes and said:

"It was as if someone had taken a rope from round my neck and I could talk again. I'm glad she's alright."

We decided not to remove anymore and Vanessa again tried talking her through the meditation.

"Try and remember what I've told you and practise every time you feel spirit around you. You will have to concentrate, but after a few tries you'll find it won't be so hard."

We arranged to visit Toni in a couple of days and after answering a few questions we left.

The next day Miriam telephoned.

"I was talking to Toni this morning and she says to tell you not to come back. If all you're going to do is make her meditate, then she doesn't want to. She can't see how that's going to stop them. She just wanted you to get rid of them all."

"We did explain to her that she would have to learn to control her own mind. With the best will in the world, we can't do it all for her - it's got to come from her. I'm sorry she feels that way, but we can't do anything more for her if she won't do anything for herself. If you remember, Vanessa told her - as I told you - it was not a quick fix and it would very likely take a year or more."

"She says she's going to find another way to sort it out - she doesn't want to wait. I understand what you said and I can see how Toni would need to get control of her mind, but she's decided it's too hard."

" I'm sorry we couldn't do it for her, but that's not the way it works. We wish her well and if you need any help with her concerning her spirit problem you've got our number?"

"Alright. Thanks for trying. She can be a bit stubborn sometimes and also a bit lazy. I'll call you if she changes her mind. Thanks."

With that, Miriam rang off. I have to say I wasn't too surprised, what with Toni living alone it would be hard to motivate herself. As she doesn't work she would have to keep her mind occupied all day and not allow herself to daydream. If her doctor had maybe consulted with a medium, especially in light of Toni's beliefs. They might have been able to overcome many of her problems by dealing with the source. Rather than medicating the symptoms. She needed a lot more determination and strength to see it through and - sad to say - there will always be some we can't help.

Case 4

Angela

I met Angela when she came to a circle I was running with Vanessa, and over a couple of weeks it became obvious that she was more experienced than most of the other sitters. On asking the president of the church, I was informed that she also did trance work. Her communication was fairly accurate and she had an understanding that newcomers didn't, although she did seem to lack confidence. This confirmed Vanessa's first assessment of her and we decided to monitor her and see how things went.

After a couple of months, while sitting with three others practising readings, Angela was taken into trance and a woman came through. We immediately saw the distress it caused Angela, so Vanessa - who was overseeing the group - helped her to regain control of the situation. Angela was very upset and explained she had been taken over before while sitting in an open circle and she was unable to stop it. We told her not to worry: we would continue to monitor her and she seemed to settle down for a few weeks.

Then while the circle was sitting together practising receiving symbols and their meanings, Angela again was thrown into trance when I asked her what symbols she had. As she looked round the circle I could see a number of spirits around her, and when she started to speak it wasn't her calm voice, but a very agitated woman who was not only loud, but very upset and frightened. I immediately went to Angela and removed the spirit, all the while talking to Angela, helping to calm her down and bringing her back into control. This caused her great upset and Vanessa took her out of the room to help her settle down. When they came back Angela was more composed but she looked worried. Vanessa explained to me that she was worried we would ask her to leave the circle.

We knew she wouldn't be able to cope with this interference on her own, so told her we would help. We decided to show Angela how to control these spirits that were interfering with her development, remove the unwanted ones, and at the same time help her to get to know a couple of her guides. To this end it was arranged that Angela would come to us the following Friday and we would help her to regain control.

Our home circle is a rescue circle and Danny, who is a trance medium, joined us to help remove the spirits from Angela, so we could talk directly to them. This proved to be an interesting evening for all concerned as we worked our way through the different spirits.

Angela's history

Before we started we asked Angela some questions to establish her history and experience with spirit and this is how it went. I asked her to tell us how she got involved with spirit and what experiences she'd had. She said:

"My mum was a trance medium. In the 1940s she and my dad were stationed in Malta and my mum would hold séances where she brought the husbands who had been killed through to their wives and families. It being a Catholic country, they had to be very careful and only hold their séances on the base behind closed doors. It wasn't until the 1950s that they moved back to England with my brother.

My father was very interested in the Indian sub-continent and their religions and beliefs, so much so that he studied meditation and trance state to the extent that he could push a needle through his hand without pain.

My brother, who was seven years older than me, was diagnosed with schizophrenia and passed to spirit about ten years ago."

"With the knowledge your parents had I'm surprised they accepted that diagnosis. Can you tell us what happened?" I asked.

"They tried to help but no-one would listen. My brother was about 19 and in the RAF. He had been hearing voices on and off for years, but he tried to keep himself aloof from everything to do with spirit. He was very outgoing and a happy person who would talk to anyone. Before he went into the RAF he had moved away from home and he would disappear for days and then just pop up again. He used to say the voices were always telling him to do things - he didn't say what. While serving, he started getting more and more upset because the voices wouldn't leave him alone. Something happened and his C.O. sent him to a psychiatrist to evaluate him and that's when he was diagnosed with paranoid schizophrenia. He was then sectioned and sent to a mental hospital and put on drugs. While he was there, he had a lot of electric shock treatments - they said it was to try and shock his brain into working properly. All that did was cause him pain, it didn't change anything, so they just kept giving him drugs to keep him docile which kept his mind dull most of the time. My parents tried to help and explain things to the doctors, but they wouldn't listen. Every time they thought they were getting somewhere, the doors were closed in their faces. After about 20 years of different drugs at stronger and stronger doses, he was put into a halfway house. Due to the cutbacks in mental health there were a lot of people who were moved out of 24-hour care and back into the community. His voice was slurred and he wasn't really aware of what was going on most of the time. I think they damaged his brain with the drugs and electric shock treatment. He ended up almost like a cabbage with brief moments of lucidity. H, he finally to a massive overdose and was found the following day by a man he had befriended. They advised us not to go and see him as his face was in such pain. He was a shadow of himself when I last visited him and he didn't know who I was. It was a terrible waste of a life. If the doctors had listened to my parents, I'm sure he would still have been here now."

"That's a real shame. It really annoys me when people won't consider other possibilities. What we're going to do tonight is remove some of the attachments you've got with you and try and get one of your guides to come through. I know you're able to meditate without distraction, but do you get spirits talking to you at all times of the day?" I said.

"Yes, it's usually when I'm doing the washing up or some other job where I don't have to concentrate."

"Have you ever experienced a loss of time - like one minute you're doing something and then you can't remember finishing it? Then you're doing something else and you can't remember starting it? Like daydreaming but more often?"

"Do you mean am I taken over? No, that has never happened."

"How well do you sleep?"

"I have horrible dreams. I usually go to bed earlier than my husband and sometimes he says he can hear me having conversations with someone in my sleep, but I don't remember.

190

Sometimes he has to come and wake me up because I'm screaming, and as we live in a flat the neighbours might think he's beating me or something. Although I wake up a little distressed sometimes, I can't remember what happened."

"You said earlier that you had gone into trance while sitting in another circle."

"Yes I was sitting in a church open circle and suddenly I went into trance and that lady who came through the other night was there - at least it felt like the same one. The circle leader helped get rid of it and then told me I had a dark energy round me and not to come back."

"Has it ever happened when you meditate or at any other time?"

"No, it's never happened at any other time, unless I'm sitting for trance. There was one occasion when a friend came over and we tried talking to the spirits. It was okay at first. My guide came through and she had a little chat. Then a nasty one came through and I couldn't get rid of it by myself - my friend had to help me. We managed to get rid of it, but it left me quite shaken. I don't have any trouble following my meditations and don't have any interruptions or anything like that and I feel very peaceful when I've finished."

Sitting for the First Time

We placed four chairs in a circle and after we sat down I said an opening prayer. We had decided not to have a meditation but to get on with what we were there for.

I asked Angela to close her eyes and ask her guide to come forward. After a few minutes I asked her if she was aware of her guide.

"I think so, but I'm not sure."

"There's a woman of about 30 with long black hair and dressed in a white tunic with you at the moment. Are you aware of her?" I asked.

"That's my guide Isabel. She was given to me by three different mediums but her hair is short now. Do you want me to see if I can bring her through?"

"No, first we have to make sure she is a guide. You say her hair was long at first, but now the one you're aware of has short hair?"

"Yes, it was about a year ago when she started to come to me with short hair."

"Why would your guide change her hairstyle? She is showing herself as she remembers herself. If her hair was never short, she wouldn't show herself with short hair. When guides present themselves to you, the way they are the first time you are aware of them, is how they will always show themselves. It's how you get to recognise them. If for instance, as in this case, she shows herself slightly differently than she has in the past, it's because it's not her. Someone is trying to impersonate her."

"Why would spirits do that?"

"Because they want to distract you and work with you. They're stopping you from learning the lessons your guides are trying to give you to help you to develop. If you think about it, your mediumship hasn't changed since the woman with the short hair has been coming to you."

"Maybe you're right, but why would my guides let her come through. Aren't they able to stop her?"

"Yes of course they are, but remember your guides can't give you bad experiences, but they can allow others who aren't guides to come through. It's all very well you getting nice feelings from your guides, but if you never experience bad feelings, how would you know when it's wrong? With practice you get to learn what is right and what isn't, but you have to recognise both sides to learn that lesson. Your guides are non-aggressive, which means if you allow some other spirit to push in front of them as they're coming through, they'll allow it to happen as a lesson for you. If you don't recognise the difference, then you aren't asserting your free will. You have to make the choice as to who you want to work with. If you choose the imposter, then that's who you'll get."

"That seems a little unfair. If I don't know the difference, how am I going to learn if they don't show me?"

"They do show you. When you meditate you say it's very peaceful - where do you think that feeling comes from? Why shouldn't it be similar when your guide comes through?"

"I see what you mean. I feel I've been taken for a ride by these spirits."

"You're not the first and there will be many times to start with when you doubt if it's your guide. I was once told by spirit 'if in doubt, chuck it out'. Your guides will always come back next time, as will the imposter, until you recognise the subtle difference. It can take a while, but if you persevere you'll start getting it right more and more until you rarely get it wrong. And when you do, you'll be able to get rid of the imposter by yourself. But the first thing we need to do is get rid of the attachments you have and then show you how to stop imposters coming through. It's only by letting them come through in the first place that you can begin to tell the difference."

"Okay. Do you want me to try again or let this one come through?"

"Let this one come through and we'll see what she has to say."

Vanessa and Danny were watching Angela closely to see if there was anything else with her.

Angela started to wring her hands and she leaned forward as though a little stooped. Then a woman came through and started talking.

"I don't mean any harm. I'm just here to help her."

"You're not her guide. Who are you?" I said

"I'm Isabel. I've been with her for a long time and I help her. I give her advice when she needs it."

"If she needs advice she would be better off working with

her guides - that's why they're with her. Don't you realise you're making it harder for her to get to know her guides by pretending to be one of them? How did you become attached to her?"

The woman started to wring her hands again and whine.

"I was told to help her. I tell her things. What are you going to do?"

"I'm going to remove you from Angela and pass you across to Danny. He will be able to keep you there safely until we've had a little chat."

I asked Danny to tune in to the woman and then told Angela to send her to Danny and to open her eyes when I told her to.

Danny nodded to me in answer to my unspoken question and I asked Angela to open her eyes, which she did.

"How are you feeling?" I asked.

"I'm okay. That wasn't my guide, was it?"

"No, although your guide was close the woman that Danny's got pushed in front. Now let's have a chat with her. Let her come through please, Danny."

"Who are you and why are you with this woman?" I asked.

"I've been helping he -r I'm one of her guides," the spirit said.

"No you're not. You're neither her guide nor are you helping. She needs to be left alone so she can communicate with her real guides. Tell me what your name is."

"My name's Isabel and I was put here with her to help."

" Will you tell me how you got attached to her please? We're not going to hurt you -we're here to help."

"What have you got covering your face?" Vanessa said.

"I have a cloth so people can't see the scars from when I was burnt. It doesn't look very nice."

"We'll make the scars go away. There, your face is healed now."

When we take away pain and scars it's our guides that help the spirit to recognise their spiritual body cannot be damaged. The spirit still has the memory of the experience they had when they were injured. Our guides just help them to understand it was their physical body that was injured, by taking away the feeling of discomfort.

"Tell us what you did to attach yourself to Angela and why," said Vanessa.

"I didn't do it - they did. They told me to stand next to her and then I sort of shifted into her energy. It was like going into a whirlpool and then I was there and I've been here ever since."

"Why did they put you there?" I asked.

"So I could live on earth again through her. As long as I did what I was told, they would let me stay."

"I see. What did they tell you to do?"

"They told me all the while I was with her, I would be able to influence her thoughts and get her to say things. They helped me to make her feel uncomfortable every time her guides came close, so she thought they weren't nice and pushed them away."

"I'm sorry but you can no longer stay with her - you'll have to leave. Don't you want to be with your family in heaven?"

"Rob's waiting for you - would you like to go to him?" asked Vanessa.

"How do you know about Rob? I've looked for heaven. There's no such place."

"Yes there is. Would you like to have a look?" said Vanessa.

"I can't. They'll get me if I try to leave and then I'll be in trouble," she said, cowering away from someone.

"We're going to put protection round you so you'll be safe, then we're going to remove the men who are threatening you. Can you see that pink haze around you?"

"Yes - is that protection? They can't get through, can they?"

"No, you're safe now, Mike's going to take you to heaven now, okay?"

"Hello again. Would you open your eyes and tell me what you can see please?"

"I can see a bright light."

"Good - that's the entrance to heaven. If you and you're friends come with me, I'll take you there."

"How did you know about the others?"

"We can see and feel them. Shall we go? Okay, what can you see now?"

"It's very bright but I'm getting used to it. I can see Rob. Can I go now?"

"Yes of course - go in peace."

Danny opened his eyes and smiled. "She was in a bit of a state worrying about getting into trouble with those men. They were throwing all sorts of feelings at her until you put the protection up."

"That's sorted. Now Angela, what I want you to do is close your eyes and ask your guide with the long hair to come forward please. I don't want her to come through - just for you to be aware of her."

Angela closed her eyes and after a few minutes it was clear she had someone with her, although she didn't let them come through.

"Now I want you let them come forward slowly but don't let them in yet. How do they feel?"

"It feels alright. I think it's my guide - shall I let her in?"

"You are aware there are others close as well aren't you? So you'll have to be careful," Vanessa said.

"I'm not aware of them. What should I do?"

"Focus on your guide all the time as she comes forward and don't be distracted by anything," I said.

As we watched we could see other spirits pushing in and a woman came through.

"Hello. I see you managed to push in then. Why're you so keen to come forward when you know we're aware of you?"

"I might have got away with it. I was made to come forward or face the consequences and I fear you less than them."

"That's a fair answer. What's your objective? Is it just to disrupt her progression or is there something more?"

"Just to work with her and have a bit of life really."

"If we were to believe that, we would be as stupid as you think we are. I didn't expect you to tell me but I thought I'd ask. How did you get attached to her?"

"I'm not. I just come and go as I please. When she works, I come and join her in case she wants to trance, then I come through to have a chat."

"I see. So you say you're free to come and go when you want, yet you just told us you were made to come through and you feared us less than them. I'm inclined to believe your first statement, as we're also aware you're not alone."

There was a shift in energies and we could feel more aggression coming from where Angela was sitting. We knew the first spirit had been removed and a stronger one had taken her place. This, of course, told us there was a lot of work to do, to help Angela to control not only who was coming through, but how to hang on to them until we had finished with them. This was the first time that Angela, as far as we were aware, had experienced our kind of set-up, where the trance medium is not in charge, but the circle leader takes control.

"Danny, can you get hold of this person and bring her through? Angela, just kick them out and open your eyes when I say so, please."

I looked at Danny and after a minute he nodded and closed his eyes and I asked Angela to open hers. Once she had settled down again, I focused my attention on Danny and who he had with him.

"Hello. What's your name?"

"Mirabelle. I'm sorry, there are some nasty men here and they make us do things to her. Can you help?"

"We will help if you tell the truth and right now you're not. Mirabelle is a funny name for a man. Let's start with the truth," said Vanessa.

"I'm a woman - there are no men here with me."

"You won't get very far telling lies. Isn't it true that you like controlling women and that's why you're here? You were really nasty to your wife and daughter when you were on the earth plane. You used them for you own ends and when they were unable to meet your demands, you beat them."

"If you say so. Anyway, what's it got to do with you? I'm my own boss and I do as I please."

"Not any longer. I've just been talking to your wife and daughter - they say you're not a bad man, just gullible and easily led. The reason you're acting tough is because your mates are watching and you're showing off. It's over for you now - you won't regain their respect, if you had it in the first place. Don't you understand they've been using you? Now that you've been caught they won't help you - they'll just stand and watch."

"Who do you think you are, as if a mere woman is better than me? You're only good for one thing and I don't need you."

"That's it - you put on a brave face, but the truth is you're tired of it all and if you could get out, you would. You care too much

197

about what those other idiots think to see common sense. Your wife and daughter are in heaven and they're waiting for you. They know it wasn't your fault and that you were ill. They still love you and want you to come home to them."

"There's no such place as heaven and you're telling lies you just guessed about my family."

"We're going to show you your family, who are waiting. Have a look," I said.

When we show the spirit their loved ones it's our guides who show them at our request.

"How did you do that? They can't be there - it's a trick."

"Don't you think you've been a fool long enough? Why would we bother to trick you?"

"Are they really waiting for me?"

"Yes - do you want to be with them?"

We could feel the energy soften as tears came from Danny's eyes and he said:

"Please can you take me to them? I'm sorry for what I've done."

"Yes of course. Just open your eyes and tell me what you see."

"I can see a bright light."

"I'm going to take you and all the others including the children who want to come. Here we are. Can you see your family now for yourself?"

"Yes. Can I go to them, please?"

"Of course. As you can see, the others are going to their families too. God bless you all."

Danny slowly opened his eyes and got a tissue to wipe his face. "There was a lot of emotion there - he really thought that where he was, that was it."

"Well at least he's home now and out of our way. How are you feeling, Angela?"

"I'm alright. I didn't think there were this many."

"I think, although we've removed some from you, there are others around the circle who are bringing spirits in to try and cause confusion. They are pushing them forward, hoping we'll think you're a lost cause and give up. We're going to try and get you together with your guides. I think we'll have to find a different one to start you off, as they're able to impersonate Isabel too easily. But that's enough for this week, so I'll say a closing prayer."

After we'd closed the circle, we had a chat about what had happened over a cup of tea. Angela said:

"I have another guide who I've worked with for quite a while will it be okay if I work with him?"

"How do you feel when he's with you?" I said.

"Peaceful and very warm inside. He's such a gentle soul. He's a monk from Tibet and he's been with me for a long time."

"That would be a good idea and forget about Isabel for the time being. Let's get you back on the right road before we try to establish contact with her again. If you play music while you're doing the housework and such, it will help to stop the chatter in your head."

Vanessa spoke to Angela the next day and she said she was fine, she'd had the best night's sleep for a long time and she was looking forward to the Tuesday night when we next sat in our development circle.

The Following Week

We arrived just in time to start the circle, so had no time to check Angela out, but she seemed to be okay. During the meditation she got a monk to join her and she had a reasonable night. We met again on the Friday and asked how her week had been.

"I've been getting on quite well. I find listening to music helps to keep my mind clear of chatter, just like you said. I've been getting sharp pains in the left side of my head just above my ear. I was going to go to the doctor's but decided to speak to you first."

"I've been getting pains in my head too, especially on Thursday, and I had a bad day," said Vanessa.

"I had a troublesome day too and Angela's face kept coming into my mind," said Danny.

"Well it's obvious you're getting interference, so we'll deal with that when we start," I said.

We started the circle with an opening prayer as usual and when we checked Angela out, there were a lot of spirits round her. So I asked Danny to describe who he was aware of: it agreed with what Vanessa was picking up, so we asked Danny to bring them through.

"Hello. What are you doing hanging around our friend?"

"I'm just seeing what you're doing, not much by the looks of it."

"That's because we've just started - perhaps we can help you."

"No I'm okay - you just carry on."

"Sorry, you can't stay here. I take it you know what's happened to you?"

"Oh yes - I'm dead, or so they tell me."

"Would you like to go and be with your family?"

"Nope, I'm having too much fun here."

"Yes, you've been interfering with our friend's head causing her pain. Well that ends now - you can't stay here. You can go to heaven, or we'll remove you and put you in a bubble of energy so you can't disturb anyone else. You'll then have time to think about the misery you've caused people and maybe change your ways."

"I'm not going anywhere, least of all heaven. I think I'll stay with her."

"Okay, we'll have to remove you. We're going to put the energy around you and send you to wait near the entrance to heaven. You'll be able to see your loved ones, but until you change your ways, you will not be able to communicate with them. When you realise your mistakes and come to terms with what you've been doing, you only have to ask and you'll be taken to join your loved ones."

Danny sent him on his way and opened his eyes. I asked Angela to focus on the monk she'd been working with in the circle the other night.

"I want you to focus until you're sure it's the right monk and ask him to come close. Don't allow him to come through - just focus on him to the exclusion of anyone else."

"I'll try. I've been aware of him for about six months now and he comes forward in some of my meditations in the other circle."

"Is he about 60 with a bald head and wearing an orange robe?" I asked.

"Yes and he comes from Tibet, I think."

"Can you bring him through, please?"

As he came through the energy changed around Angela and we all knew it wasn't a monk. I asked Danny to draw him away from Angela and after a few moments Angela came back, as Danny brought him through.

"You knew you weren't going to fool us, so why did you come through? You've been impersonating her guide for a while now, haven't you?"

"Very clever aren't you? Well, what do you want? I'm a busy person."

"We just want to stop you from interfering with our friend's development. You can go to heaven and be with your family."

"There's no such place as heaven so I'll stay here."

"You know Maggie's waiting for you, don't you," Vanessa said.

"How do you know about Maggie? You're reading my thoughts, aren't you?"

"First, if I was reading your thoughts you would have to be thinking about her and you weren't, and second I can't read thoughts. I'm talking to her - she's in heaven waiting to see you."

"Really. Then what does she look like?"

"I'll do better than describe her - I'll show her to you. There - can you see her?" Vanessa said.

"Yes that's her. How did you do that?"

"It doesn't matter. You now know I'm not reading your mind. You can be with her and the rest of your family if you want. You only need to say so and we'll take you to them."

The man's face fell, as he was obviously realising that he'd been betrayed by those around him into thinking there was nothing else, and the things they'd got him to do.

"I would like to go and join them if I can, please."

"Of course you can. Just open your eyes and tell me what you see."

"I can see a bright light, but I've seen that before and that's how I met this lot and I've been with them ever since. They're not very nice, you know."

"We know. We're having them removed now by our guides. If you look over there you'll see another light, but it's not as bright."

"There's lots of lights. How is anyone supposed to know which one is right?"

"By the feeling you get from it. Come into this light with me and see the difference."

"It's peaceful and calming. I see what you mean. I can see my wife and son. Can I go now?"

"Yes of course," I said.

"Sorry for the upset I've caused. Thank you for your help."

Danny opened his eyes and smiled.

"He was very apologetic when he realised what he'd done. I could feel him cursing himself for being such a fool."

"He'll be alright now. Angela, there's an Indian woman standing next to you. Do you know of any guides from India, because I feel she is a guide?"

"I don't know of any. Do you want me to try and tune in to her?"

"Yes, see if you can sense her and tell us what you're getting, please."

After a few minutes Angela started talking.

"The lady is about 50, quite small with a small diamond in her nose. She's got one of those saris on and she's bare-footed. Shall I bring her through? She makes me feel very peaceful."

"Yes, let's have a chat with her," I said.

She came through gently and spoke in a soft voice. There was no agitation or discomfort from her in any way.

"Hello. Can you tell us where you come from, please," I said.

"I come from India a long time ago."

"How long ago?" I asked.

"About 3000 of your years."

"How long have you been with the lady?"

"Since before she was born. I have been trying to help her, but she wasn't listening to me. Those others were more forceful and she only heard them."

"She does have a monk and a lady called Isabel as guides, doesn't she?"

"Yes, but because she has been led astray by those others they will step back until she is ready to greet them again. Hopefully a valuable lesson has been learnt."

"Yes, I think so. It's a good reminder for all of us. Thank you for coming to talk to us. Can you bring yourself back now, Angela?"

After Angela had come back, we decided to close the circle and closed in prayer.

"That was really nice. She is a guide, isn't she?" asked Angela.

"Yes she is and when you meditate or ask for a guide in future, ask for her. Don't accept anyone else. You know what she feels like and what she looks like. Remember and always look out for any differences before you let her through next time. She will always look and feel the same, okay?"

"Yes. Thank you all for helping me to get rid of those imposters."

"It's not over yet. Let's see how you're getting on next time we meet," I said

The following Tuesday when we arrived at the circle Angela was looking a lot less tired and quite enthusiastic.

"I've had a good week with no chatter and a decent night's sleep so I'm looking forward to getting to know my Indian lady a little better tonight," she said, in answer to my question as to how she was.

Throughout the evening I kept an eye on Angela and she seemed to be doing fine. Her clairvoyance was accepted and she was quite cheerful. Afterwards I asked her how she felt.

"I've had a good night and I'm not feeling apprehensive about going into trance. I feel more in control now."

"Its early days yet - let's keep an eye on things to make sure you have everything under control. We'll give it a couple of weeks and then we'll sit again and see how you're getting on with the Indian lady," I said.

"That would make me feel better, knowing you're keeping an eye on things. I really don't want to get in that situation again. You don't think I'll have any more trouble, do you?"

"We hope not, but it's best to be sure," said Vanessa. "As Mike said, it's early days yet. There's still a lot to understand and we need to build your strength. Then you can control the nasty spirits if they try to come through again. Rest assured, they'll try and they'll succeed to start with but with practice and guidance you'll be able to overcome them."

"We want you to get to know at least two guides so you can get used to the different feelings your guides give when they come to you. It will help you to see the difference between your guides as well as the others," I said.

Angela seemed satisfied with that, and having no more questions, we said our goodnights and left.

On the next circle night we arranged to turn it into a fledgling evening, so the sitters would gain experience standing in front of a group of people. During the interim period, Angela got a lot of voices telling her she was useless and not to bother going to the next circle as she wouldn't be able to do it - she wasn't good enough. Playing music only stopped it for a while, she said, when I phoned her during the week and she told me. I told her to ask her guide to come close and help her to ignore the voices and to focus on her Indian lady. When we met on the Tuesday, Angela said it had helped and got better as the week progressed until today, when it got louder and more insistent, but she was still managing to hold her own.

I checked her out and she seemed quite calm and peaceful, so I just kept an eye on her during the evening. When it was Angela's turn she stood up and calmly gave her evidence and message, which was understood with no trouble at all, and she sat down again after she had finished.

When we had finished the evening, I asked Angela how she felt and she said:

"Once I got up, the voices stopped as I tuned in to my guide and asked for a communicator. Once I was aware of the communicator, it was as though there was no-one there but me, him and the recipient. All I did was focus, just as you keep telling us."

"It would appear you're starting to get things under control, so we'll just keep an eye on you for a while to make sure you're okay."

Angela has had no problems for the past two months and she now has two guides she knows and works with.

Finally

These are just a sample of the cases we have come across where people have been diagnosed with schizophrenia, MPD, or DID. As you can see, some can be helped and some can't. It's dependent on the history of the person and their strength of mind as to whether we, as mediums, are able to help or not. If the person is on medication it's less likely we can help, because they tend to rely on medication for relief instead of strength of mind. There may also be underlying reasons for their medication that are not obvious. We are not medically trained and would never recommend that people stop their medication because they have spirit interference. There are a number of causes for hallucinations - sleep deprivation, alcohol and drug abuse to name a few; there are also side-effects from some prescribed medicines. All that goes on when someone is being haunted in whatever way, can be overcome with guidance and strength of mind, and an understanding of what's happening and why. I have visited hundreds of houses over the years; most have known it to be spirit interference, and it has been cleared satisfactorily once the people involved understand what's happening. Most don't have any interest in the spirit world - they're just in the wrong place at the wrong time. Sometimes people just move into a house where there is a lot of spirit activity. There are many reasons why some houses are haunted and others aren't. There are some who bring the problem on themselves by playing with things they don't understand, like the Ouija board. A lot of people get spiritual problems when they have a traumatic experience, which can heighten their awareness. Once they've become sensitive to the spirit world they usually have problems controlling it. After we've explained and given them an understanding of why it's happening to them, we're able to clear them or their home and they don't have any more problems.

We also as mediums are able to talk to the spirits and help them to understand what's happened. Most of them don't realise the affect they are having on the home or the people in it. Once they realise they are usually very apologetic and move away from the house to continue their journey in the spirit world.

It's unfortunate that the medical profession are not able to accept the possibility of interference from outside the body, i.e. discarnate spirit. If they were to refer suspected interference cases to a medium, at least they would have considered all possibilities before prescribing mind-altering drugs. To give a diagnosis of any of the schizophrenias, MPD or DID, can be a mind-blowing experience - literally. They should try to put themselves in their patient's place: being told you have a mental disorder can completely change your perspective of the future and your place in it. I myself was diagnosed with Parkinson's disease about three years ago and that was bad enough; there was a lot to come to terms with. But to be misdiagnosed as schizophrenic, MPD or DID as a lot are, can have such an effect that there have been cases where people have taken their own lives, rather than put their family and themselves through the misery and difficulty of the future.

There's a great responsibility on the part of the medical profession and scientific community to look into all aspects of the conscious and subconscious mind. A greater understanding would stop many misconceptions of what is, and what isn't, a debilitating disease and give many people peace of mind. I know research costs money, but there is an untapped resource of mediums all over the world who could help put things in perspective. If only the scientists and medical profession would open their minds to the possibility that not everything is of this world. When they realise the brain and the mind are separate but closely integrated, only then will they begin to understand what mediums have known for years - that man is a duality. Can you imagine the great leaps forward, the understanding of who we really are, and perhaps the repercussions on the religions of the world? When they realise we're all from one place, there will be no more wars.

Glossary of terms

BPD - Bi-polar disorder.

DID - Dissociative Identity Disorder.

MPD - Multiple Personality Disorder.

HAUNTING - where a person is aware of a ghost.

SPIRIT OR SOUL - the divine part of the self which is eternal, containing all of the experiences and knowledge of past lives.

DISCARNATE - without a physical body.

SPIRIT GUIDES - spirit beings who assist us in our spiritual work.

SPIRIT WORLD - Heaven.

SPIRIT REALMS - a place between heaven and earth where spirits are sometimes lost.

SPIRIT ATTACHMENTS - where spirits sometimes merge with the aura or energy of the individual.

TARDIVE DYSKINESIA - a condition marked by involuntary movement of the tongue or facial muscles, especially after long treatment with phenothiazine tranquillizers or similar drugs.

PROTECTION - an energy similar to a force field that is put around the house and or person by our guides.

ASTRAL BODY AURA - the astral body is invisible to most: it is an ethereal substance that interpenetrates the physical body and extends to about 7 inches.

CLAIRVOYANT - the ability to see into the ethereal realm without using physical eyes.

CLAIRAUDIENCE - the ability to receive sounds, words, sentences and voices, with no apparent source.

CLAIRSENTIENCE - the ability to perceive information by a feeling within the whole body without outer stimuli related to the sensation.

CIRCLE - where mediums sit to learn to develop their mediumship.

READINGS - when a medium gets communication from loved ones for a sitter.

Recommended reading

Psychiatric Drugs Cure or Quackery by Lawrence Stevens JD
Schizophrenia a Non-existent Disease by Lawrence Stevens JD
Stay away from Psychiatrists Warns by Lawrence Stevens JD
Psychiatry under fire www.thegaurdian.com.news/mentalhealth
Death Rates from psychiatry are rising www.pyshc.central.com/schizophrenia
Psychiatry should be abolished www.antipyschiatry.org/abolished
Successful Schizophrenia www.successful schizophrenia.org
Schizophrenia Breakthrough by Al Siebert PhD Practical psychology press
The Resiliency Advantage by Al Siebert PhD Practical psychology press
The Survivor Personality by Al Siebert PhD Practical psychology press
Brain Damage: Psychiatry's Legacy by Gene Zimmer sntp.net/brain
Causes of Schizophrenia en.wikipedia.org/wiki/schizophrenia

Bibliography

Collingwood, Jane. Premature death rates rising in schizophrenia, bipolar
patients. (2011) [Online] Available psychcentral.com/lib/premature-death-
rates-rising-in-schizophrenia. [Accessed April 2012]

Doward, Jamie. The Observer Psychiatry under fire. (12 May 2013) [Online]
Available http. www.thegaurdian.com.news/mentalhealth. [Accessed Sept
2013]

DSM-1V Diagnostic and Statistical Manual of Mental Disorders: (2014)
[Online] Available from sntp.net/reference/dsm [Accessed Feb 2013]

National Institute of Mental Health: Causes of schizophrenia (circa 2013)
[Online] Available from: www.nimh.nih.gov/causes-of-schizophrenia
[Accessed June 1012]

Siebert, Al PhD Practical psychology press. Brain disease Hypothesis for
schizophrenia disconfirmed by all evidence (1999) [Online] Available from
www.SuccessfulSchizophrenia.org/articles/ehss/html

Siebert, Al. PhD. Schizophrenia breakthrough. (nd) [Online] Available from
www.practicalpsychologypress.com [Accessed Jan1012]

Siebert, Al. Phd. The Resiliency advantage. (nd) [Online] Available from
www.practicalpsychologypress.com [Accessed Jan 2012]

Siebert, Al. PhD. The survivor personality. (nd) [Online] Available from
www.practicalpsdychologypress.com [Accessed Jan 2012]

Stevens, Lawrence. JD. Psychiatric drugs: Cure or quackery (nd) [Online]

Available from. http:sntp.net/drugs/quackery.htm
[Accessed 10th Sept 2013]

Stevens, Lawrence. JD. Schizophrenia: A non-existent disease. (circa 2010)
[Online] Available from. http:www.scribd.com/doc/35068144 [Accessed
Sept 2013]

Stevens, Lawrence. JD. Warns stay away from psychiatrists. (circa 2012)
[Online] Available from. http:www.examiner.com/article/lawrence-
stevens-jd. [Accessed Sept 2013]

Steven, Lawrence. JD. The case against psychotherapy. (nd) [Online]
Available from. http:www.antipsychiatry.org/psychoth.htm
[Accessed Sept 2013]

Zimmer, Gene. Brain damage: psychiatry's legacy. (nd) [Online] Available
from sntp.net/brain-damage/brain

Printed in Great Britain
by Amazon